CRACKDOWN

CRACKDOWN

SURVIVING AND RESISTING THE WAR ON DRUGS

GARTH MULLINS

DOUBLEDAY
CANADA

Doubleday Canada and colophon are registered trademarks of Penguin Random House Canada Limited

Library and Archives Canada Cataloguing in Publication

Title: Crackdown / Garth Mullins.
Names: Mullins, Garth, author.
Description: Includes bibliographical references.
Identifiers: Canadiana (print) 20240380843 | Canadiana (ebook) 20240394674 | ISBN 9780385674898 (hardcover) | ISBN 9780385674904 (EPUB)
Subjects: LCSH: Mullins, Garth. | LCSH: Addicts—British Columbia—Vancouver—Biography. | LCSH: Recovering addicts—British Columbia Vancouver—Biography. | LCSH: People with visual disabilities—British Columbia—Vancouver—Biography. | LCSH: People with albinism—British Columbia—Vancouver—Biography. | LCSH: Heroin abuse—British Columbia—Vancouver. | LCGFT: Autobiographies.
Classification: LCC HV5805.M85 C73 2025 | DDC 362.29/3092—dc23

The poem "Hundred Block Rock" is reprinted with permission from *Hundred Block Rock* by Bud Osborn (Arsenal Pulp Press, 1999).

Cover and text design: Andrew Roberts
Cover image: Elaine Brière
Typesetting: Terra Page

Printed in the USA

The authorized representative in the EU for product safety and compliance is Penguin Random House Ireland, Morrison Chambers, 32 Nassau Street, Dublin D02 YH68, Ireland. https://eu-contact.penguin.ie

Published in Canada by Doubleday Canada,
a division of Penguin Random House Canada Limited,
320 Front Street West, Suite 1400,
Toronto, Ontario, M5V 3B6, Canada.
Distributed in the United States by Penguin Random House LLC.

penguinrandomhouse.ca

1st Printing

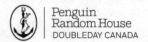

Penguin
Random House
DOUBLEDAY CANADA

This book is dedicated to our many fallen comrades,
too many to name, killed in the long drug war.

It is also dedicated to my partner in all things,
Lisa Hale.

Contents

Nick's Funeral

We all knew how Nick died. But nobody talked about it. By unspoken consensus, his cause of death was not to be mentioned. We wanted to show sensitivity to the family, who were in full-blown denial, yet even amongst ourselves, we talked in whispers. Our crew had lost nearly a dozen from overdose.

Hundreds of others were dying of overdose in British Columbia. The Health Board had recently declared a public health emergency. Activists had put one thousand white crosses in Oppenheimer Park to memorialize the dead. I knew that the "China White" heroin going around was dangerously strong, but I'd never get through the funeral without some. Before I left the rooming house where I lived, I did a big smash. Now that I was here, the dope in my system was just something else to feel anxious and guilty about.

We gathered on the sidewalk out front of Glenhaven Memorial Chapel under a holiday-brochure-blue sky, a rare sight in terminally grey Vancouver. Cars and trucks rumbled past. A siren screamed along East Hastings Street. Friends and family nodded acknowledgements to each other, chatting and smoking before the service got started. There were a few jackets and ties, but mostly jeans and hoodies. I was wearing a plaid work shirt and had shined my boots to try to show some respect.

We made our way inside the small chapel, and I picked up a program from a table by the door. It was the standard Glenhaven layout, produced for loved ones too shell-shocked to choose fonts and colour schemes. Across the front of the program was a portrait of Nick with "Celebration of Life" written underneath in flowery script.

I found a seat on a pew near the back. There were mumbled syllables, the odd cough and shuffle of feet. Tinny speakers dispensed church music that sounded like it was recorded on a 1980s-era Casio keyboard. Nick's mother, father and younger sister sat up front, near the casket, where Nick was laid out in a suit jacket and tie. I'd never seen him wear anything other than T-shirts and sneakers.

The pews were filling up with punks, skaters and metalheads. We all partied, went to shows and played in bands together. Weed, MDMA, acid, mushrooms, cocaine and binge drinking were common. Sometimes even a little speed. But heroin? The few of us who used it kept quiet. We knew that junkies were considered the lowest of the low—bottom tier in the fuck-up hierarchy—beneath drunks, cokeheads and even glue huffers.

In the months before his death, Nick had made some changes in his life. He wasn't partying as much and had started vocational training—something to do with computers. He'd put on a few extra pounds, as you do when you kick dope. He had a healthy glow. Then one night he relapsed. Maybe he wanted to celebrate a recent accomplishment. Maybe he felt depressed. Or maybe he was just bored. Whatever his motivation, his tolerance was low from all those months of not using.

The music stopped. An officiant provided by Glenhaven took his place at the front and cleared his throat. The chapel fell silent, and he started his speech. I could tell he'd given it before because he only paused to check his notes when mentioning Nick's name. I drifted in and out of his spiel, recognizing bits of bible verse from past funerals. It was like an old top forty song on AM radio that I didn't especially like but took comfort in its familiar lyrics. The Nick I knew was no Christian, but I guessed his parents were. It wasn't my place to judge.

In a pew two rows ahead, my ex-girlfriend Nina turned to look at me, and I could feel judgment simmering inside her. Nina was tanned and outdoorsy. She was a vegetarian and did yoga. She was spiritual and saw magic everywhere. We went hiking, camping and swimming together. I thought she would save me from myself and my habit. With her, I'd be someone new—someone good.

At the front of the chapel, the officiant continued his speech: "He leadeth me in paths of righteousness . . ."

But instead of becoming someone new, I was sneaking off to shoot dope in Nina's bathroom while she cried. Eventually, Nina asked, "Why do you love heroin so much more than you love me?" I had no answer. It was never her job to save me. She had her own problems. Now, two pews ahead, I could tell she knew I was still using. I wished I could disappear.

"Yea, though I walk through the valley of the shadow of death," the officiant continued.

Up at the front, a baby began to fuss. Nick's girlfriend rocked the bassinet, and the cries subsided. The baby had never met her father. Nick's parents had only met their granddaughter for the first time that day. They looked shattered. I could feel Nick's mom starting to unravel.

One by one, we made our way down the aisle to pay respects at Nick's open casket. Ahead of me, someone exploded into howls of pain. When it was my turn, I looked down at Nick's body. He was lying there in his suit, with his hair pulled back, his eyes closed and his face expressionless. Whatever spark had animated Nick was gone forever. I wanted to stay with him. I put my hand on his. It was cool and dry. "I'm sorry," I whispered.

Nick's parents stood nearby, accepting condolences. As our crew worked its way past, I could feel Nick's mother radiating waves of grief—and something else too. Anger. Resentment. Blame. I wanted to say something comforting to her. I wanted to tell her that Nick was a smart, funny and self-effacing guy. That he had been a genuine friend to me and to so many others. I wanted to hug her and tell her how sad I was. But I couldn't say anything. The same drug that killed her son was now circulating in my bloodstream.

I felt implicated in Nick's death, the dope in my system an insult to his memory. I had to get out of here. Outside, I looked for our friend Ashley. I could tell she blamed herself—she'd been with Nick on the night of his death, and now I was worried that she might hurt herself. When I found her, I asked if she was okay, but she couldn't speak. I lit a smoke and passed it to her. She hugged me and cried into my chest. She would never be the same, carrying that misplaced guilt with her until she herself died, a few years later.

My old roommate Liz walked up. "I can't believe he's gone." We hugged, then she pulled back, appraising me critically. She knew. "Do you want to die too? Like Nick?" Heads turned to look. "Haven't we lost enough friends? You're smarter than this." She was shaking her head. "Don't be such a selfish asshole."

"I know, I know," I said. Nina was standing just behind Liz. She had been listening, and now she stepped forward. I thought she was going to join in, that I was about to get an impromptu intervention from the whole crowd. But Nina didn't say anything. Big tears started rolling down her face. This was much worse. Liz continued, "When are you going to get clean?"

I didn't know.

"I'm sorry. I'm sorry," I said, trying to edge around the crowd. I felt unworthy of their concern. I promised to quit, I promised to get help. I promised anything to get away from these people who cared about me.

I needed dope. Now.

I walked a few blocks west on Hastings until I heard a familiar voice. "Rock? Down?" I recognized the dealer. I scored a couple of points of heroin, folded up in flaps of discarded lottery tickets. I stepped into an alley to fix. Using outside was not fun, but it was a way to keep safe. If I overdosed, someone might see my body and call the paramedics. Maybe I wouldn't end up like Nick.

I pulled up forty units of water into my syringe and dumped both points into the barrel. I shook the rig, found a vein and inserted the needle. I pulled back the plunger just enough to see a drop of my cold, dirty blood flag in the clear solution. "Goodbye, Nick," I whispered as I pushed the plunger down and the drugs flooded my system.

I looked up. Sun shone through a jumble of electric cables, transformers and telephone lines that snaked down the alley, held aloft by ancient wooden power poles that formed big H's. The heroin rolled through my bloodstream. My breathing slowed, my heart calmed. I let the drugs wash away the guilt. I tucked my syringe carefully back into the glasses case I kept it in.

Heroin killed Nick, but I needed it to live.

PART 1
GETTING
WIRED

Distant Early Warnings

Bundled in layers, I stood in our backyard, the ghost of my breath rising into the dark January evening. Sometimes I could hear the northern lights crackle, and I wanted to capture that sound on tape. My family's pet Samoyed, Anouk, stood beside me. Through my mitten, I thumbed the red record button as two glowing bands of green undulated across the night sky.

The little machine whirred as the cassette's take-up reel started turning. I'd heard from other kids that if you whistled at the aurora borealis, the lights would swoop down and snatch you away. If whistling was dangerous, what about recording them?

Back inside our house, I kicked off my boots, hung up my parka and shut off the tape. The dog's wagging tail thumped the wall. In the warm kitchen, Mom, still in her office turtle-neck, stirred chili con carne in a lime-green electric frying pan. I played my recording back, but there was no crackling aurora. Just the sound of me and Anouk breathing.

Yellowknife sits on Dene land on the northern shores of Great Slave Lake. It was built around two gold mines, on the edge of the arctic treeline, and wore a stubble of stumpy jack pine, dwarf birch and black spruce trees, punctuated by lakes and outcroppings of glacier-scored rock. It seemed like it was almost always winter.

My family lived in a house for government workers, with red-and-gold shag carpeting, a basket-weave fence and a giant sunflower that sprouted each summer. My parents moved north for work in the territorial government. Other southerners came north for work as miners, teachers, nurses or bush pilots. It worked out well for southerners; not so much if you were Indigenous.

The townspeople were into country music and disco, gold ore and Labatt 50, skidoos and bush parties. Our phone number was only five digits, and a special dinner for us was a bucket of Kentucky Fried Chicken, the only fast-food joint in town. All the boys I knew wanted to be miners, hunters or hockey players. But I didn't know what I wanted to be, only what I couldn't be.

Gold was the unofficial religion. There were gold bars on the flag of the Northwest Territories, and on the edge of town, the Con Mine's Robertson headframe stood as the tallest structure in the Territories. It squatted over a deep mine shaft, lowering men down and hauling ore up. I used to imagine the miners following the gold veins as they tunnelled under the town, hollowing out the earth. In the sandbox, I tried to dig my way to join them.

A group of locals even wrote and performed a musical called *Two Hands and Forever* as an ode to the rugged individualism of the northern prospector who dreamt of a never-ending gold strike, two hands wide, running through the Precambrian rock forever. Practically the whole town, including my family, went to see it in the high school auditorium. A chorus of miners and musicians sang:

> *My dream is of tomorrow,*
> *And when I fill my pockets with gold,*
> *I'm gonna stake my claim,*
> *And write my name in letters big and bold.*

I loved the winter, but those long dark nights gave most adults the long dark blues, which many treated with alcohol. The booze made adults unpredictable, at one moment celebratory, the next angry, and children had to read what mood was filling a room on any given night. Drinkers who felt unwelcome or were barred from the Gold Range bar often drank outside the post office on Franklin Avenue. Some to numb out southern pasts; others to numb northern colonial traumas. Fingers and toes lost to frostbite marked the daily battle of forgetting.

But drinking was only considered a problem if it stopped you from getting up for work in the morning. Drinking was often part of the job, part of most workplace cultures and part of the fabric of the town. Hard work was true north on the family compass, affirmed by generations of soldiers, loggers, mill workers, schoolteachers, shop clerks and distillers. And my parents.

When the snow finally melted, the winter's lost mittens, wrenches, planes—and sometimes even lost people—resurfaced. In the brief camera flash of summer, we all burst out of our houses, plants shot up out of the earth, and horseflies swarmed out of the muskeg. On June and July evenings, the sun stalled low over the horizon, only dipping below for a couple of hours.

It never got dark. The long, warm summer days were photo negatives of winter. I loved the languid evenings and how they slowed down and stretched out like hot road tar. Adults got strung out on sunlight, and kids played in the streets past midnight. Dad put tinfoil on our bedroom windows to simulate night.

My father was a tall, confident and athletic man, full of postwar optimism and restless energy. He had a stoic, self-reliant quality, and nothing seemed to rattle him. I wanted to be just like him. I didn't know what he did at his office job, but I knew he could make furniture, portage a canoe, gut a fish and fly a plane. He had a bush pilot's knack for navigation, planning and observing weather. He showed by example what it was to be a man. It's what he wanted for me. And I wanted to be that way for him. But things that seemed to come effortlessly for Dad didn't come so easy for me.

In the summer when I was seven, Dad and another pilot strapped our aluminum Grumman canoe to a six-seater Cessna 185 on pontoons and loaded a week's worth of food into the cargo hatch. My mother, my sister, Anouk and I all climbed aboard. We flew over an endless tundra dotted by lakes too numerous to have English names. Up front, Dad and the pilot had agreed on one of them, and landed on the still water. We unloaded onto the shore, and Dad unstrapped the canoe.

After the pilot took off in the float plane, we didn't hear another engine or see another person for a week. But there were bears, wolves, fish and bugs. Lots of bugs. Mom and Dad loaded the supplies into the canoe, then we all got in. Dad sat in the stern, with a compass around his neck and waterproof map case against his plaid shirt. Mom paddled from the bow, in her orange rain poncho.

Mom and Dad's paddles dipped rhythmically across clear lakes. I thought about how big everything was, and I asked Dad how long it would take to count to one trillion. "Many, many lifetimes," he said. We were so small out here, but Dad was confident and competent. He knew everything. "Look at me when you're talking to me," he said gently, trying to teach me to fake eye contact.

We camped on little islets made of dinosaur-ancient rock spackled with lichen and colourful flowers the size of pinheads. We fished for northern pike and Arctic grayling. Dad cleaned them on the shore, letting the guts roll into the lake. Mum cooked the filets on the fire. We all slept in a tent, with my sister, the shortest, sleeping at the end. The land was ancient and vast beyond comprehending. I felt at peace with everything.

The midnight sun, down near the horizon, was warm. It couldn't hurt my eyes or burn my skin. Small waves lapped on the shore. A loon's note-bending call echoed across the giant quiet at the top of the world. I carved its silhouette into the lichen with my pocket knife, then lay on my back on warm rocks and looked up into the dome of the sky: blue at the edges fading into violet fading into indigo and black. I held on to the rock. I could fall straight up, into space, into the black forever and be gone. If I just let go.

My arrival had overwhelmed my parents. As a newborn, I couldn't open my eyes. I had no pigment in my skin, hair or irises. I had albinism. "We expected a perfect baby," Mom later told me. "All our friends seemed to have perfect babies."

At home, I rocked in my crib, banging my head on the wall and cracking the plaster. Doctors called it a "rhythmic movement disorder"—a self-soothing habit common among children with low vision. I kept my eyes closed, or squinted. When they were open, my eyes danced around, never still.

My parents didn't know anything about albinism, and no one offered any support. Even their friends pulled away. Mom said she felt alone. They researched my condition, and found a parents' group, where they saw children frightened to leave their parents' side. Mom didn't want me to be like that. "I wasn't a cuddly mommy. I pushed you out because I was so concerned about your ability to cope." As a toddler, I was scared to lose track of her in crowds. I felt a distance between us.

At first, I couldn't distinguish anything from anything else. I couldn't make out faces looking at me. The world was too bright, blurry and shaky. I didn't speak.

As I grew, I learned to identify objects by snatching images out of a vague, overexposed mess. I could see an oval and recognize it as a head. I could make out contrasting areas—eyes and hair. But I couldn't see the colour of the eyes or the expressions on the face. Focusing on an object took effort. It almost hurt. And after a few seconds, my eyes would glitch out and jerk away. Eventually, I learned to wrestle patterns out of the impressionistic chaos. I had to be ready to jump when those patterns were disrupted, or resolved into something bad. *That blob might be a bus. That blob is coming toward me.* I paid close attention to sounds and the feelings in my gut, chest and throat.

Patterns emerged from continuity, repetition, relation or interruption; from an intake of breath, or an extra beat of silence; from a little change in pressure or temperature. A room seems to get colder when it contains rage. The barometer drops when someone is trying to hold back their feelings. If I can't make something out, I have to wait. Time reveals patterns.

I got a magnifying glass at school—the kind they sell at the pharmacy. It wasn't nearly adequate—but in Yellowknife it was what they had. I remember at one parent-teacher night, Dad didn't mumble when he used the word "albino" in conversation with a teacher. He was not ashamed of me. He enunciated the syllables with defiant neutrality, as if challenging the teacher: "There's nothing to see here. My son is not a freak." But I also overheard Dad sharing a bleak vision of my future. He worried to my mom that if I didn't work hard and overcome my disability, I'd grow up to be lonely and unemployed, spending my days smoking and watching bad TV. He wanted me to try to overcome my weaknesses—to defeat them—not to be a victim.

Our dog guarded me while I napped and taught me to walk, holding one of my hands gently in her mouth as I staggered up and down stairs. I learned to navigate our house in the dark. I knew all the walls and corners, not just from memory, but from sound. Every space whispers its own intimate tone, if you listen. The hum of the fridge reflecting off the window. The sound of the wind outside, being muffled by the carpet. The ticking of a clock down the hall reverberating off one wall, then the other. Each tiny source is a sonar signal, bouncing back to me and forming a picture in my head. Sound was to be the main way that I understood and related to the world.

For my birthday, Dad made pancakes and gave me a bike. "Better a few broken bones than a broken spirit," he said. I wiped out a few times, once leaving a four-inch gash down my leg. But I loved it. "Boys don't cry," he said. That turned out to be good advice in a northern mining town.

So I pedalled all over Yellowknife with a small battalion of grade-schoolers from New Delhi, Tuktoyaktuk, Sheffield, Red Deer, Abbotsford and Dettah. We had snowball fights and bike races. We pretended we were on Hoth, the ice planet from *Star Wars*. All the boys wore the same jeans, plaid shirts and North Star sneakers that came from the one clothing store in town. We smoked cigarettes and shared beer pilfered from our parents. We hung out on a dilapidated dock on Frame Lake and paddled around in a canoe we found there. During spring breakup, we jumped from the shore onto the ice pans. It was freedom.

But I couldn't see well enough to be a hunter, hockey player or a pilot, and the word "albino" set me apart from my friends. I hated the sound of it. It was an iceberg word—cold, with submerged meaning. Reptilian, pale and androgynous. I was embarrassed by the rhino-piano-beano sound: Al-bine-oh. A lab rat. A red-eyed rabbit. An exotic snake. A psycho-pinko, white-whale movie villain. A blind, colourless cave-dweller. A snowy ghost. A reptile ghost boy.

I'd later learn that my parents wanted to have another child, but the doctors warned them off. They told them it was likely their next kid would also be born with albinism. And they said it was morally irresponsible to knowingly inflict that kind of handicap on another child. My parents followed the advice of the day and adopted my little sister, Gill, rather than risking a repeat.

After lights out, I would sometimes lie awake, listening to a blizzard howl outside. With eyes shut tight, I saw a snowstorm of blood-red dots, swirling against an endless black field. The light photons that drowned my eyes during the day still danced at night. My pulse whooshed in my ears. I turned on the radio for company. Sad cowboy songs that made me feel better. Then the weather forecast in English and Dogrib (Tłıchǫ Yatıì). A list of cold temperatures in remote villages: Hay River, Igloolik, Norman Wells, Inuvik, Great Bear Lake, Port Radium. I remembered what my Cub Scout leader, Akela, had said to all his little charges that day in the church basement: "We cannot allow the north to become a home for deviants!" After CFYK signed off for the night, I rocked back and forth on lullaby waves of soft static. *Am I a deviant?* I wondered.

The Lack

loved Yellowknife, but southwestern British Columbia had stamped itself into my parents' souls. Northern winters were too long and too bleak. So we packed the yellow station wagon and left for Vancouver.

My life changed radically when we arrived. The city scrolled out forever in every direction. There was no edge that I could find. No wild spaces without adult regulation. I was nine, and not supposed to roam outside of a box formed by the four main streets around our house.

On my first day at school, I realized Vancouver kids had sophisticated tastes. They talked about the brands of their sneakers and jeans, while I had generic Yellowknife clothes, uncombed hair and Coke-bottle glasses, along with a small-town accent and the wrong slang. The kids didn't bike, fish or explore like they did in Yellowknife. Instead they played team sports. In gym class, baseballs, dodgeballs, handballs and other spherical sports objects would careen out of the fuzzy distance and smack me in the head.

My school in Vancouver seemed further ahead academically than we were up north. Compared to the other kids, I couldn't read or write property or do multiplication. I sat in the front of the class but could never get close enough to actually see the blackboard. In grade three, the books mostly had big block letters, but the text got smaller in grades four and five. I hunched over the books like a gargoyle, trying to get close enough to see.

Once a kid hid my magnifying glass before a test. I couldn't see where he put it, but I could tell by the snickers around me that everyone else knew. The exam started and the teacher ordered me to sit down. Instead, I flipped my desk over and walked out. I failed the exam and was sent to the principal's office. But I didn't snitch on the kid. School authorities rarely had the patience to hear me out and didn't believe me anyway. Why would I appeal to them? I knew I had to fight my own battles.

"You just aren't trying," my homeroom teacher told me. I stared at the bottle of Aqua Net hairspray she kept on her desk. My mere existence seemed to inconvenience her, and she resented any small accommodation measure. If I didn't have to copy everything out by hand from the textbooks, "it would be unfair to the other kids," she said. Mrs. Aqua Net suggested I'd be better off at a "special school."

Kids called me snowman, Billy Idol, whitey, Casper the Ghost. And, finally, just Ghost. In grade six, some of the boys decided that I was also gay and ridiculed me with homophobic slurs. "Hey, Ghost. What'd you do this weekend? Drive the Hershey highway?" One kid liked to chassé across the classroom, holding his hand up in a hateful little pantomime, then break into an Eddie Murphy routine: "Hey boy, you look mighty cute in those jeans. Now come on over here and fuck me up the ass."

———

One of the good things about being in Vancouver was that we were close to my extended family: my grandfather, my great-aunt Rose and my uncle Wayne and aunt Sandra. Rose's family moved from Hong Kong in the 1960s, and marriage brought them and the Mullinses together. At family dinners, we would gather around a big round table at my uncle's. Rose would always make my favourite dish: chicken corn soup. She and I were close.

For my tenth birthday, my grandfather gave me a shortwave radio receiver. He and Dad slung a long wire high over a neighbour's tree for an antenna. Grandpa knew all about this stuff. He was a radar technician with the RCAF in World War II. When he got home, he built the first television in British Columbia.

When I flicked the switch, the planet's radio signals bloomed in my orange foam headphones. I filled up my logbook with signals from around the globe: Radio Moscow, BBC World Service, Voice of America, Radio Netherlands and dozens of other stations. There was a massive world humming out there beyond the blocks I was allowed to explore. I tuned in to lonely ham operators transmitting from the Mojave Desert or from an Arctic research station. They made me feel less alone. I imagined myself not just listening but broadcasting to the world one day.

My friend James was into shortwave and electronics too. We sat together in class and hung out after school. James and I repaired old televisions so we could watch TV in our bedrooms, without parental monitoring. We salvaged old surplus army radio gear, soldering and wiring up a secret phone network so we could talk at night without our parents overhearing. James helped me build a stereo system out of spare parts and garage sale finds. At the school auditorium, he showed me how to run a PA and mix live sound.

My grandpa told me to use my words, not my fists, so that's what I did. I talked myself out of most scraps—and into a few. I never started a fight, but I never ran from one either, and if a friend was getting bullied, I had their back. Yet whenever I got hit by another kid, it happened fast and I'd be seeing stars before I knew what was going on. Soon, I started to recognize the pre-conditions. The sound of a group of boys laughing derisively made me change my stance. When one broke off from the group and approached, I'd put my weight on my back foot. I'd keep just out of range and face the kid side-on. It made me a smaller target, gave me better balance and let me strike, if I had to. I turned my body into a sensitive antenna, tuning in to the faint signals of oncoming aggression. I wasn't much of a fighter. I lost most—but not all—of them.

My class followed Terry Fox's Marathon of Hope. He was running across Canada to raise money for cancer research. Kids brought in newspaper clippings and Mrs. Aqua Net rolled out a big TV. We all sat cross-legged on the floor to watch coverage of a young, curly-haired Terry Fox running down the shoulder of a highway on a prosthetic leg. Passing cars honked and waved. The kids fell silent as we watched. I could hear the class hamster, running on its little wheel. The principal talked about Terry Fox on the PA that morning. He said Fox was inspirational for "overcoming his handicap" and "pulling himself up by his own bootstraps." Overcoming is what Dad wanted me to do. But the marathon only made me feel worse. If Terry Fox was a hero, I was a zero. I wasn't overcoming anything or inspiring anyone.

After Mrs. Aqua Net rolled the big TV away, she sent me to the school's basement, which smelled of orange peels and hot dogs. Down there was a room called the Learning Assistance Centre, or LAC for short. Kids called it "the Lack," as in lack-of-brains. Metal mesh covered the windows, cutting the outside world into little squares. Upstairs, advanced pupils went to the Learning Enrichment Centre, proudly adjacent to the principal's office, full of sunlight and shiny new computers. No bars on their windows.

Once a week I was sent here to meet with Mr. Manzer, a social worker with a beard and glasses from the Department for the Visually Impaired at the Ministry of Education. I was never keen to talk about my albinism or blindness. I didn't want people to think of me as a complainer. But I wondered if Mr. Manzer had some answers. He wasn't blind, but he worked with kids across the Vancouver school system who were.

Mr. Manzer showed me how to wash my dark-tinted, scratched-up Coke-bottle glasses. My eyesight was so bad that I hadn't noticed how dirty my lenses were. He showed me how to comb my hair and wash my face. He asked me questions about life at home. "Do you have trouble finding your clothes in the morning?" I didn't. "Do you brush your teeth before bed?" I did. Mr. Manzer quickly realized I needed something a lot stronger than the weak magnifying glasses I was given at school. He gave me a loupe, a high-powered magnifying glass for jewellers. I hovered it a couple of inches over the page, bending to meet it like a giraffe drinking at a watering hole, and dragged sentences through the thick lens, one word at a time.

Mr. Manzer then showed me a big electronic reading machine called a VisualTech. It was like something from NASA's Mission Control. I put a book on a tray under a camera, and enlarged text appeared on a screen. The machine was not portable. You couldn't curl up with a novel in bed. You had to sit at a workstation in the Lack and feed literature into the machine's eye.

Mr. Manzer suggested I try using a white cane, but that was a step too far: I already looked like an alien. I knew the cane would make me an even bigger target. Was I supposed to adorn myself with all these devices until I looked like a cyborg?

When Mr. Manzer asked how I was feeling, I didn't know how to answer. I didn't have the words to say that I felt ashamed or humiliated. Or lonely, even among classmates or family. I didn't think of myself as suicidal, I just didn't want to exist. But I couldn't tell him that. I carried my feelings around deep in the pit of my stomach. Hidden even from myself. I saw the patience and compassion he had for me and I was grateful. Mr. Manzer never rushed me. And he never blamed me when I was slow.

Then, at one of our weekly meetings, Mr. Manzer handed me a bus pass. The Canadian National Institute for the Blind issued bus passes to all members. It was my ticket to freedom. He even took the bus with me a few times, showing me how to navigate the transit system. Finally, I could escape from the little box that contained my school and house.

At night, I put on a hoodie, grabbed my bus pass and snuck out the window. I caught the number 22 and rode the whole route, hoping to disappear into the strange city. The bus drove through sleeping residential districts. The beach at night. Burrard Bridge over dark water. Empty lit-up office buildings in the downtown core. Neon Chinatown. From the west side to the east side, from Burrard Inlet to the Fraser River. My anxiety dissipated in the warm diesel rocking of a cocoon bus on a rainy night. The world was full of people awake at two a.m. Night after night, in transit but going nowhere, I vanished among a nation of night owls, relieved that this city also held eccentric misfits, not just kids in the right clothes.

But the bus route looped around on itself. It always led back home. And it always led back to her, to Victoria. I didn't know it then, but my life would keep looping back to her.

No Future Now

Mr Manzer had suggested I attend an alternative program at a local high school where he worked. It was supposed to be for students who got good grades, but also for kids who didn't do well in big institutional schools. So that's where I went.

The hallways were full of jocks and teenage yuppies, scrubbed, moussed and gelled into pastel and neon forms that smelled like Obsession or Brut 33. In Benetton tops, jelly bracelets, acid-wash jeans and shoulder pads, they listened to tooth-achingly saccharine radio hits. There were also burnouts, metalheads, nerds, artists, gangsters and skinheads. I didn't really belong to any group. I would have called myself an outsider, but I didn't know there was an outside.

Everyone looked forward to getting their driver's licence. In all the movies, the guy picks up his date in a car. But I was too blind to drive. The high-performing students were rushing toward their futures, making plans for university, business, travel, marriage and babies. I was pretty sure I wasn't going with them. I felt like there was nothing to look forward to.

Our school had its own version of DARE—Drug Abuse Resistance Education. Nancy Reagan yelled "Just say no!" loud enough that we could hear her clearly in Canada. Cringey after-school specials starring Scott Baio, Burt Reynolds and Michelle Pfeiffer reinforced the anti-drug messaging. Everyone mocked them. Soon after Ronald Reagan declared a new war on drugs in the US, Canadian prime minister Brian Mulroney jumped on board. Mulroney announced that "drug abuse has become an epidemic that undermines our economic as well as our social fabric."

One day we had a special guest speaker. "You think this is funny?" a tough-looking guy asked, pointing at all of us sitting in our uncomfortable little desks, the kind with the seat attached to the table by a metal bar. I drove my knee into some sharp-edged part underneath, to dispel anxiety. The guest speaker seemed sincere, even though his tough-talking, scared-straight routine was court-ordered.

Michael and I sat next to each other, as we did in many classes. We were friends. Michael often read to me off the blackboard or explained things—like algebra or chemistry. My printing still looks like his neat draftsman's characters. As the sermon picked up speed, we both sunk down in our seats, hoping the guest speaker wouldn't notice us. His message was too late for me.

I was not getting good grades at school. I was not on the road to becoming the man my dad wanted or the student my mother had hoped. Somewhere around age twelve, I just said "fuck it" and started sneaking out at night to bludgeon all my anxieties and self-hate to unconsciousness. I wanted to smash it all to black. I raided Dad's supply of generic beer in stubby bottles. I siphoned off some Red Tassel vodka from a twenty-sixer kept in the kitchen cupboard. I bought pot and hash off the local mulleted weed dealer. The school's anti-drug education wasn't going to rob me of that relief.

In the back of the class, a couple of the kids giggled. "Don't drop the soap," one whispered to the other. The special guest speaker turned to glare at them. "Prison is no joke. None of you would last one hour." Then his tone dropped down, quiet and confessional. When he was sixteen, he killed his abusive father and had been in trouble ever since. He warned us about the perils of drugs, shoplifting and dealing, and about violence and rape in prison. The class was silent, even the soap gigglers. Everyone looked at their desks.

We all got it. Drugs equals jail. Jail equals rape. There was no useful information imparted. Neither the guidance counsellor nor the guest speaker told us about HIV/AIDS. BC's right-wing Christian premier, Bill Vander Zalm, was against AIDS education for students.

It was a deeply conservative time. Ronald Reagan and Margaret Thatcher's Cold War triumphalism and free-market fundamentalism were like wallpaper. "There is no alternative," Thatcher had repeatedly scolded those who longed for anything other than capitalism. This is it. There's nothing else. Greed is good. It's just human nature. Dreaming of another world is silly. This is the best world possible.

After the anti-drug lecture, I met up with Janet. Janet was a punk who marched the halls of our alternative school in big biker boots. She took me under her wing. Janet was four years ahead of me—and she was pregnant. But she never tried to hide her baby bump, and she never took any shit for it either. I wished

I was as courageous as her. I looked forward to seeing her when we'd hang out at lunchtime or on rare occasions when she'd take me to her place to listen to music after school.

One day Janet gave me a dubbed cassette copy of *London Calling* by the Clash. The title track is a reference to the old BBC World Service station identification, "This is London calling." I plugged in my headphones and hit play. Kick drum, snare, distorted guitar stabs and then—Joe Strummer sings in an English accent about police violence, nuclear meltdown and drug users nodding out. I played the whole album twice without stopping.

I never realized that music could hold so much meaning. Finally, something real. This was the signal that I'd been longing to receive. The Clash led me to the Ramones, Dead Kennedys, SNFU, NoMeansNo, Circle Jerks, D.O.A. and more. The lyrics championed underdogs with chantable slogans and biting satire. I learned about Harvey Milk, Pol Pot and the Spanish Civil War. I sang along to anthems against sexism and racism, against Reagan and Thatcher and even against Bill Vander Zalm.

Punk gave voice to a vague but urgent feeling bubbling inside me, a desperate need to escape but with nowhere to escape to. Everything was bullshit and nobody was coming to save me. The music felt like a personal message. It wasn't just me who was fucked up. Everything was fucked up. It was such a relief.

My dad said, "Why do you like this music? It's so negative. These people are losers. They have no future." I wanted to disagree, to pull out lyrics sheets and point out deft political critiques. But it wasn't just the politics that drew me in. Punk's nihilistic, futureless, fuck-the-world side spoke to me too. I wanted to change everything. Including myself. But I also wanted to destroy everything. Especially myself. I knew my dad wouldn't understand.

Punk gave me style. Having bright platinum hair was no longer a mark against me. It was perfect. I cut it into a spiky flattop and strapped on a pair of surplus combat boots. In a subculture full of skinny, pale kids with dyed hair, I fit right in. Punk camouflaged my albinism. I could own my own outsiderness. I walked down the street with a new kind of defiant swagger. People had always stared at me, but now I'd give 'em something to look at.

I started to go to alternative clubs like Luv-A-Fair, also known as Scuz. Cocktails were ninety-nine cents. Nine Inch Nails, the Subhumans and the Violent Femmes played there. I was tall for my age but I still needed a fake ID. Behind Spartacus Books, a guy with a laminator would crank out a "BC Identacard" for any kid with ten bucks. It didn't work everywhere, but it did the job in enough cases.

After-hours clubs like Heaven and the Industrial Eclipse were all-ages. They played alternative dance music: Ministry, the Cure, New Order, Skinny Puppy and the Smiths. A spinning disc of light beams cut through the fog to Johnny Marr's tremolo guitar intro on "How Soon Is Now." The dance floor filled as Morrissey's lonesome wail soothed our teenage angst.

It was at these places—not at high school—that I met girls. At Heaven, a twenty-two-year-old woman hung out with me most of one night before she asked me how old I was. "Thirteen," I said sheepishly, knowing she was about to leave. "Go home, it's past your bedtime," she laughed.

Another night I was so drunk I kept burning myself with my own cigarette while slumped against a wall behind the DJ booth. Natasha, a girl with a giant mohawk, took pity on me and brought me home. She was a couple of years older than me, and everyone seemed to hold her in respect and awe. We started dating.

After the clubs shut, Natasha and I would go for breakfast at a twenty-four-hour greasy spoon with a crew of our friends. Debriefing over eggs and coffee after a long night was always the best part. Sometimes we'd jump the fence of an outdoor public pool, night swimming and yodelling bad Morrissey impressions as the sun came up. Since the last bus was long gone, I'd walk home, hopefully getting there before my parents got up for work and noticed my absence. At school I slept through classes with my head on the desk. Other times I skipped altogether.

To fund this life, I worked a series of jobs. I was a lighting and sound technician for local schools putting on plays and musicals. I babysat for friends and neighbours. My uncle hired me at his construction company. I worked for a moving company, did phone sales and took odd jobs off a board at the unemployment office.

Back at school, a jock with a surly, mush-mouth way of talking and a blond military haircut had it in for me. He hated my guts on general principle. There was an army of these guys whose mission it was to rid the world of freaks. Several grades above me, he thought he was Iceman from the movie *Top Gun*.

"I'm gonna kill you after school," he hissed at me in the hall-way. But now I had older kids from outside of school on my side. A gang of them showed up for me just as this meathead was about to kick my ass behind the corner store. They chased him off.

I graduated from schoolyard fights to the real kind, with adults. I was six-foot-four by now, and there was always some real-man asshole wanting to scrap. One night on the 321 bus, a grown man with a mullet punched me in the face because he thought I was gay. Another time, in the parking lot of a 7-Eleven, a group of guys cornered me. "Fucking AIDS junkie," one said. The leader took me down with a kickboxing boot to the head. The rest piled in with jabs, kicks and haymakers, while I curled into a ball on the ground. I stumbled away and blacked out. A friend found me and took me to the hospital, where I was told I had bruised ribs and a concussion. "Don't fall asleep tonight," the doctor warned. Violence was every-where, like a background hum.

I was still going to school but living part time with Natasha in a three-storey walk-up apartment with half a dozen punk kids. We'd hang out on the Granville strip. There were two-dollar smoke shops, a cheap repertory movie theatre, endless refills of burnt coffee, 25-cent peep shows and a bowling alley under the sidewalk. A harmonica busker on the corner of Robson and Granville always honked out the same riff from an old blues song, ending with a little walk-up turn-around, then starting back at the beginning, endlessly repeating. For years and years, I never heard him play anything else. Some of our friends had squatted in a burnt-out sex shop. Everyone who stayed there smelled like a campfire. Adult predators drifted among the kids. An older guy hung out behind the Burger King. He'd pay five dollars if you'd kick him in the nuts. I never did.

I did my best to avoid the monster-size skinheads. They had names like Chainsaw, Razor and Fifi and stomped up and down Granville Street. Some of the skinheads seemed to just love fighting. But others were part of small fascist militias like Aryan Resistance Movement (ARM), White Aryan Resistance (WAR) or Church of the Creator. A far-right leader had even gone to my high school. Years later, Tony Mac admitted that his group had a cache of guns for the "racial holy war."

There were gigs at the Smilin' Buddha Cabaret, IWA Hall and the New York Theatre to raise money for political causes. Punk woke me up to politics and the idea that you can fight back. I wanted to meet other people who were worried about the same things as I was. I wanted to be part of something. I searched out anti-fascist meetings and demonstrations against nuclear cruise missile testing. I started a group at my high school called Student Peace Activist Movement, SPAM for short.

We held meetings and fund-raisers, and formed a coalition with other groups. Our first big action was to organize a flotilla to try to stop a US nuclear warship entering the harbour. One of the other students had a sailboat. Or his dad did. At five a.m., we motored out to the middle of Burrard Inlet and waited. Our motley collection of Zodiacs, canoes, dinghies and kayaks arranged itself into a nautical picket line. Local communist organizer Charles Boylan piloted a tiny inflatable that he'd modified to look like a pirate submarine. Cops watched us from their own speedboat.

Peering through binoculars, I spotted a massive grey hulk emerging from the fog. "¡No pasarán!" crackled over the marine radio from another boat. I raised my binoculars again. The distance had closed rapidly. The aft quarter of this ten-storey ocean-going leviathan filled the lenses. I could easily make out a dozen sailors in white dress uniforms, standing beside a pair of deck guns. One was waving.

The warship roared right through the flotilla. The calm sea was churned into large swells and white foam. Some smaller boats were swamped. In the chaos, the cop boat crashed into the communist submarine. Kayaks and canoes helped stabilize and right each other. As we tied the sailboat up dockside, a reporter pushed a mic at me and asked what I'd hoped to accomplish. Taking off my lifejacket, I said, "I don't want politicians to blow up the world while I'm just getting to know it."

Back at school, the PA squawked to life. "Garth Mullins to the vice-principal's office, please." The vice-principal had seen the news coverage and received complaints from parents. He was angry. He ordered our peace group to disband and threatened to suspend me. "Focus on your studies," he advised. Instead of being in trouble for my own failures, I was in trouble for leading a righteous cause. We didn't stop the warships, but I realized that fighting back felt better than doing nothing—even when you didn't win.

While some of my classmates were full of optimism about their future, I could see none for myself. As people planned adult lives, I was getting dragged home by the cops. But by some small miracle, I graduated from high school, although it seemed my grades were not good enough for university. I imagined myself working in radio or electronics, as my grandfather had. Maybe I would go to a trade school. But I didn't feel enthusiastic about any of my options. More and more, I relied on booze and drugs to avoid thinking about the future or about myself. I was drifting toward the bleak life my dad feared for me. But I told myself not to care. I wanted to be a rebel who refused to conform. But I felt like a reject who had never been invited to join in the first place.

The Headframe

looked out the window into painfully bright whiteness. It stretched from horizon to horizon, covering the tundra like a new blanket. I closed my eyes and turned away. In a plane full of mineworkers, I was among the youngest, at seventeen. I thought about the long shifts in an isolated mining camp. Six weeks on, two weeks R&R, repeat. Working mining meant being apart from my girlfriend, Natasha. It was a dry camp, so I worried about having no booze or drugs to use to escape from myself. I felt anxious about flying into abstinence. But the money was good and included food and accommodation. Plus I had no other prospects. Plenty of northern kids worked mining after high school. I'd never thought I'd join them, but the head of Echo Bay Mines wanted to give opportunities to disabled people. The plane landed on the snow-packed airstrip and taxied to a stop. There was no turning back now.

A ground worker popped the hatch, and the cabin filled with arctic air. Outside, the omni-whiteness was interrupted by a series of buildings connected by metal tubes, all painted in International Orange—a colour designed by some safety committee to set objects apart from their surroundings. It's the colour of cold-water-immersion survival suits, the Golden Gate Bridge and space shuttles' external fuel tanks.

We trouped down the plane's stairs and to a building where Ted, the head of security, met us. In a crewcut and black military bomber jacket, Ted x-rayed and searched our luggage. He was the thin blue line to prevent booze and drugs from coming in, and gold from getting out. This far north, there were no cops. The company was the law.

In the break room, there was a bulletin board with safety notices. A sign on the wall warned:

NO INSUBORDINATION.

NO STEALING.

NO FIGHTING.

NO INTOXICATION.

NO SLEEPING ON THE JOB.

INFRACTIONS RESULT IN IMMEDIATE DISMISSAL.

I was given a safety briefing and then assigned to the mine mill. Crossing one of the catwalks, I got a good look. The mill was a screaming cacophony of rock-smashing, limb-crushing machines and mad-scientist chemistry on an industrial scale, all wrapped in kilometres of pipes, cables and conveyor belts. There were a thousand ways to die here.

Ore was mined underground and taken to the mill to be crushed, ground, aerated, leached and filtered. Then gold—and a little silver—was recovered and poured into glowing bullion under the watchful eyes of Security Ted. Everything else was tailings: heavy metals like zinc, lead, arsenic, cadmium, cobalt, mercury and tonnes of pulverized waste rock were pumped out through pipelines to form huge lakes on the tundra, the beautiful landscape of my childhood.

Every day at seven a.m., I reported for work at the mill planning office, where I'd do paperwork or wait for one of the bosses to send me off to various jobs around the mine site. I could be seconded to any team or work by myself for days. Student hires like me usually got the boring jobs nobody else wanted to do.

I worked all over, cleaning up a graveyard of broken mine machinery on the old airstrip, organizing the tool crib, assisting with maintenance on mill machinery, painting loader scoop buckets in bright Caterpillar Highway Yellow, welding, torch cutting, picking up garbage and filing.

For a few weeks I worked with the tailings pipeline crew—Stu, Dave, Kevin, Kuz, Henry and Doug. We laid down kilometre after kilometre of pipe, installing heat trace wire so the tailings didn't freeze up, insulation and aluminum cladding. We'd argue about what music to put on the boom box. Rush? Whitesnake? Metallica? Bob Marley? At least everyone agreed on my Clash tape.

Near the end of a shift, in twenty-four-hour daylight, I was assigned to take tailings samples with a worker from the environmental office. We got the sampling gear, jumped in a pickup and headed out to the tailings ponds. On the horizon, the tundra started rippling, and the landscape itself came alive with caribou. The Bathurst herd of some 350,000 animals was migrating in a big arc across the Arctic. The caribou filled the road. We had no choice but to kill the engine and wait. I was transfixed. The cab was filled with dust, the musky smell of ungulates, the sounds of grunting and stamping hooves. We sat in silence as thousands of animals passed by over the next half hour. Some of the herd stopped to drink from the tailings ponds. I sadly pondered why the company couldn't build fences around the toxic lakes to keep the animals away. I wrote it all down in my notebook and vowed to keep an eye out for future opportunities to change things.

After a long shift, I'd open the meat-locker door to the ATCO trailer I shared with a farm boy, a metalhead and a group of geologists. I'd flop into my bunk and sleep like the dead. The white noise of mill machinery, like radio static, pushed me under.

The hard work and long hours took their toll. Decades of mining could wear you out, and I could see it on the lifers. The guys who worked here were separated from their families by hundreds of kilometres. Some had injuries from previous accidents. Some had been exposed to chemicals or radiation from uranium mining. It was a hard life. There was little fighting here, since we all had to live and work together and nobody wanted to lose a good job over some petty beef. After working twelve-hour shifts, most people were too tired anyway. Within a week or two, I'd made a couple of friends and knew the site pretty well.

There was a fraternal, pumped-up masculinity. The bullshit and banter was often peppered with homophobia and misogyny—though the four or five women who worked at the mine wouldn't take shit from anybody. But there was something else too. The brotherhood in this remote place was a way to check in with each other. We're all okay here, right? I can count on you? We relied on each other to keep safe. I was proud to be part of it.

At the back of the mill, there was a hole in the floor, a shaft dropping a mile down to the bottom of the mine. The mill was room temperature but the ground just under it was permafrost, which caused steam to corkscrew out of the hole, lit yellow by sodium vapour lamps, shining up from below. It looked like the portal to hell. The 7:15 a.m. cage popped out of the steam, hauled up by creaking cables that ran up to the drum hoist in the headframe.

A dozen of us tagged in and boarded: an Alberta bronc rider, an Inuit father and son, an engineer with a tan, a couple of hard drinkers drying out on their second day in, and the two geologists I was working with. The drone of the mill faded as we descended. Rock walls sparkled with ice crystals as we passed through the chill of the permafrost layer. Deeper, the thermometer crept back up to about ten degrees Celsius—the body temperature of the earth's crust. The broken rock emitted a damp, primeval smell. The mile-long journey down took eight minutes.

The cage stopped at 950 metres down. The geologists and I disembarked and turned on the lamps on our hard hats. We waited for scalers to clear a section of the drift, knocking loose rocks off the ceiling so they didn't fall on anyone. Then we entered. The geologists looked at their clipboards and spray-painted borehole sites and angles on the rock face. Directions to follow the gold vein.

The diamond drillers, paid by the metre not by the hour, were impatient to get going, to sink holes that would be filled with explosives, to blast the drift further into the rock, chasing the gold vein. Then the smoke would clear and the process would begin again, repeating twenty-four hours a day until the deposit was played out. Then on to the next strike. Gold fever.

In the silence, some whispers carried along the drift to me. A couple of guys were talking about cocaine. I had wondered how people managed with no booze up here. Now I knew. But I doubted they'd risk their jobs by selling any to a newcomer like me.

Like many mines, Lupin was a dry camp. This was for safety reasons, the company said. But Yellowknife had mines and bars. Mineworkers there went to the Gold Range for a few beers at night and reported for work the next morning. Up here, the sameness of every day and the enforced sobriety was getting to me.

I got bored. I got homesick. I got restless. I got lonely. There were two hundred people on site, but depending on your shift and assignment, you sometimes worked, slept and ate by yourself. Hearing protection to mitigate the tumult of machinery put you in a kind of sonic isolation for hours, alone with your thoughts, occasionally communicating by screaming directly into a co-worker's ear or via pantomime: thumbs up for okay, two fingers to the lips for a smoke, a middle finger to say no thanks. I counted the minutes until morning coffee. Then lunch. Then afternoon coffee. Then until the end of shift. I counted the days until the two weeks' R&R, until the end of my contract. I needed a vacation from this place. I needed a vacation from myself. How do I find the guys with the coke?

People couldn't smuggle in booze. Security Ted and his x-ray machine would find the bottles right away. They needed something stronger and smaller in volume. I'd later learn this was something called the Iron Law of Prohibition, a term coined by economist Richard Cowan. He said, "The harder the enforcement, the harder the drugs." And enforcement at Lupin was pretty serious about booze. But this didn't stop mineworkers from wanting something to take the edge off after a twelve-hour shift, or something to help get through the long arctic night. So people smuggled in weed and coke. And probably other stuff that I didn't know about. If they had just let people have a couple of beers after work, there wouldn't have been as much of an underground market. Mineworkers wouldn't have to risk getting shitcanned, or a record that would blacklist them from the whole industry. If you got caught, you'd be on the next plane south.

After the snow melted and the temperature warmed up, I went fishing with the pipeline crew out on Lake Contwoyto. We caught some Arctic char and cooked them using caribou antlers for a grill. I said, "A couple of beers would go down pretty good right about now." Bob pulled out a joint. I'd found weed pretty boring down south, but up here it was perfect. At least to me. Bob fired it up and passed it around. I thanked him profusely, and we all laughed. It was the best joint I've had in my whole life. Bob was now my weed guy. We'd smoke up behind pallets of lime in Cold Storage #2.

But Bob flew out for his two weeks off, and I was back to sobriety. I had no choice but to try to make it work. Maybe I would feel better if I thought of this as my decision rather than enforced abstinence. I cut out coffee and smokes, since it's pretty hard to have one without the other. I read books about meditation and Buddhism, trying to find my sober Higher Power. I walked out onto the tundra, sat down and tried to think about nothing for twenty minutes a day. In the endless Arctic desert, my brain instantly filled with regrets, recriminations, cringing embarrassment and moments of shame and mortification. I quit trying to meditate after three minutes. I was no zen master.

At work I was getting on really well with Jack. He was a tall, skinny guy too. He had some kind of pigment irregularity that made his skin blotchy, but I couldn't see it. Maybe he felt a kind of kinship with my albinism. Like most full-timers, Jack was on a two-weeks-in, two-weeks-out rotation. But it wore on him. "Every time I go home, it's a different month," he said. "At home, everybody's coming and going, doing their thing. Not me. I'm not in sync."

When Jack was back home in Alberta, he asked me to fill in for him. After two weeks he came strolling back into the office, ducking his head around. He looked down at the paperwork, twisting his millwright's ring. "Congratulations. Seems like you didn't fuck it up." He offered advice about getting on full time. A permanent job wasn't a bad option. I loved the land. But if this was to be my life, I needed to learn how to stay sane up here.

So I kept going back to my meditation spot. The Arctic hares noticed me, noses twitching, keeping their distance and skittering off if I moved even slightly. I tried to be still, finding it impossible. But then I could do it, for a moment. Over the next few days, the hares got closer. In my third week, a calmness came over me and a brave one edged up to me and put its paws on my leg.

I did this every day, the same drove of Arctic hares keeping me company. In the massive stillness of the tundra, in its haunting beauty, I was momentarily okay. But whenever I got back to the mill, I was still terrified to be sober and alone with my ghosts.

I dreamed of dying out here. Not tragically or violently, just a day without a tomorrow. To disappear, having never existed. Buried in the Barrenlands, the lichens slowly colonizing my bones over millennia. Peaceful. I didn't want adulthood. I wanted nothingness. Oblivion.

Coming in from the tundra, I unwittingly walked under a burst pipe leaking a lead nitrate solution. Between my hearing protection and the din of machinery, I couldn't hear it splashing onto the concrete floor from high up in the mill. I only knew something was wrong when I felt burning. I ran to an emergency shower, pulled the chain and washed it off. In less than a minute, the plastic of my hard hat had melted and I had chemical burns on my neck.

This was a dangerous place for anybody, but especially a blind guy. I quit meditating. What was the point? I was good at some aspects of the job, but I needed to find a safer line of work or risk getting seriously injured. I wrote letters of appeal to the post-secondary schools that had rejected me for having bad high school grades. I told them I had low vision and promised not to take math or any of the other subjects I'd failed at high school. The University of Victoria offered me a shot.

The days got shorter. The last of my contracts ended, and I caught the company plane to Edmonton along with the outgoing shift of mineworkers. I've never seen a more thirsty crew. We stormed the airport bar, my co-workers trying to blunt their re-immersion into the civilian world. Bob bought the first round of boilermakers for the pipeline crew. He handed me a pint, dropped in the whiskey, and sloppily banged his foaming glass into mine. "Let's get wrecked!" he hollered. The bar cheered back. I was going to miss these guys.

Locked Up with Inspector Gadget

Slam! There was an all-too-familiar noise outside. The sound of a cop car door banging shut is unmistakable. We all recognized it. Nothing else on earth sounds like it. We were scouting out an abandoned building as a possible squat—but nobody wanted to catch a trespassing charge.

"It's the cops," I whispered. "Run!"

The three of us took off in different directions. I hid in the brush. My heart pounded and insects rustled while police searched along the road. I slowed my breathing and thought about how I got here.

A couple of friends and I had driven down to California from Canada on a spontaneous, low-budget road trip. Just a few months before, I was working at the mine and then living in Victoria, taking classes at the university. I was shooting coke, using meth, MDMA, pills and whatever else I could get my hands on, but I didn't have a habit yet. I was always searching for something, and I thought maybe I'd find it down Interstate 5. But now I was running from the law.

After what seemed like hours crouched in the brush, I figured the police must have given up. I poked my head up and looked straight down the barrel of a shotgun, levelled at me by a big-necked cop in aviator sunglasses. He was pissed off at having to waste his time looking for me.

"Get out of there. Down on your knees. Hands behind your head. Interlace your fingers," he barked.

"Yes, sir." I snapped into institutional compliance mode.

"Failure to follow orders will be considered resisting."

"Yes, sir."

The gravel on the road bit into my knees, but I didn't move. The cop snapped the cuffs on tight, placed me into the back of the cruiser and threaded the seatbelt through the handcuffs. The cops caught my friends too.

At the cop shop, a booking officer filled out paperwork and took my fingerprints and mug shot. "Turn to the left." My belongings were inventoried and put in a big zip-lock bag: Timex watch, grey-and-black hat, earring, broken red pocket knife, plaid lumberjack coat and seven cents cash. My boots were seized for evidence. Once the booking officer had all my belongings, he made a thorough search, going through each pocket and feeling the seams. After a few minutes, he read me my rights again, this time for drug possession.

When I was placed into a packed holding cell, someone immediately asked, "What time is it?" There were no cigarettes, no windows and no clock in here. It was a room out of time. Guys lay on the bench or paced the small floor space in varying (and conflicting) states of agitation and relaxation, intoxication and detoxification. Arguments flared up and died down.

The next night, a bus came for a group of us. It drove out of the city. Buildings disappeared and arid farmland spread out in all directions. After some unknown amount of time, the bus rolled up to a sprawling complex. We were unloaded and strip-searched. The intake officer issued me with a "felony red" jumpsuit with "Monterey County Correctional Facility" stencilled on the back, my first clue about our location. I was also given a plastic drinking cup, toothbrush, disposable razor, thin plastic mattress, scratchy blanket and beige plastic sandals that made running and kicking next to impossible. The intake officer snapped a plastic bracelet around my wrist with my inmate number printed on it.

It had been over a day since my arrest, and I was looking forward to lying down. A CO walked me and a half-dozen others through corridors and sally ports, dropping us off at various places along the route. Nobody was yelling "fresh meat" like in the movies. New arrivals were a mundane daily occurrence.

I was deposited in a large, echoey room designed to house sixteen prisoners, but there were twenty-seven of us in there that winter. A bunch of three-tier bunk beds had been brought in to accommodate the overcrowding. Four octagonal metal tables were bolted to the floor, with four metal chairs attached to each. This was my pod. The fluorescent lights were dimmed, and most people were still asleep. It felt like it was around five a.m. I found an empty bunk, rolled out my mattress and flopped onto it.

A skinny, middle-aged white guy with a scraggly beard strolled up, smoking a cigarette rolled so tight his cheeks caved in with the effort of getting a drag. "You're in the wrong place," he said. Prisoners had divided the pod. There was an invisible boundary, splitting it in half. Black prisoners on one side, Latino on the other. A few whites in the middle. When I arrived, I had randomly put my bedroll in the Latino area. Now I was being ordered to the white zone.

Scraggly Beard's crabby hand extracted the tiny smoke from his mouth and I caught a glimpse of faded ink. Was that the arm of a swastika wheeling out from under the sleeve of his uniform? Was he Aryan Brotherhood? I was new here. It showed, and I knew it. Squinting at this guy's tats to determine prison gang affiliations would probably get me an ass-kicking. So I shifted my gaze.

"I'm good here," I said. I started to realize that bunking out-side of the segregated areas was dangerous. I knew if I wasn't with some group, I'd be vulnerable on my own. But in my gut, I knew I wasn't safe anywhere near this guy. For now, I left my bedroll in the spot I'd chosen. Scraggly Beard looked back at the white-guy bunks, then at me. He shrugged, as if to say, oh well, it's your funeral.

A couple dozen glasses of milk had been set out on one of the metal tables. I helped myself, drinking one down in a sin-gle long pull. "That ain't yers," Scraggly Beard scolded from his bunk. I looked at the empty plastic cup in my hand. It had three black burn marks in a row along the rim. My prison-issued cup was still on my bunk. The remaining full cups all had various burn marks and scratches, each one a unique pat-tern identifying the owner. I'd only just got here and already drunk somebody else's milk, snubbed a potentially dangerous Nazi and flouted the bunk segregation norm. This wasn't going well.

I lay back down and tried to sleep. *How the fuck am I going to survive in here?* I thought. I'd only shut my eyes for a few minutes before Scraggly Beard came sauntering up again. I could feel him looming over me, so I opened my eyes and sat up.

"It's my turn to mop the pod today," he announced.

"Oh, yeah?" I mumbled.

"Not no more!" he replied, almost giggling. Scraggly Beard swung the mop handle toward me and gestured at it. "When it's my turn to mop the floor," he said, "you're gonna do it." I was too tired to do anything but acquiesce, so I stood up, pulled up my red jumpsuit, slid on my beige plastic sandals and took the proffered mop. I started swabbing the deck, mopping around the metal tables and past the two pay phones for outgoing calls.

Not far from the phones were three toilets and two showers. Whatever you did in them was visible to all. One wall of our pod was thick glass. There were identical pods below us and across from us. More tiers of pods radiated out in spokes from a central hub. From the air, the building, one of a dozen, must have looked like an asterisk. COs could watch everything in all the pods from an observation tower in the centre. It was the same panopticon design that had been used in institutions like this for ages. Everyone had to eat, shit, scheme, shower, play cards, read, call loved ones, ferment booze, pray, network, bullshit, watch TV, sleep, argue, make crafts, tattoo, fight and fuck in full view of the guards and everyone else.

I mopped my way across our pod in slow, lethargic circles. Scraggly Beard called out instructions that he found hilarious: "Missed a spot! Put yer back into it!" I was reminded of my uncle, whose construction outfit I worked for one summer, giving me instructions on the correct sledgehammer technique. "Let the hammer do the work," he said. I made wider mop arcs, letting my hand slide down the handle, the way I learned to swing that sledgehammer.

"C'mon, get moppin', Garth," Scraggly Beard shouted. This was immediately misheard by someone, who exclaimed, "Poppin' Garth? Who's that? Are you 'Poppin' Garth'?" My nickname was born and quickly passed through the pod. "The new guy is called 'Poppin' Garth'." This was immediately abbreviated to P.G., which had a double meaning, since I was the youngest prisoner on the pod, something not lost on one massive guy who sat on his bunk brooding. I could feel his predator eyes on me as I worked.

I mopped my way over to the TV. There was only one, which could be turned off at any time by the COs in their tower. They used it to punish us, and so that we'd punish each other. Turning off the TV was used as a weapon against people who weren't even watching it. If anyone's behaviour caused the TV to be shut off during *Dance Party USA*—interrupting Ice-T, Prince or the Beastie Boys—there'd be hell to pay. This was the only music in the pod.

A big guy was planted in front, watching the TV intently. He had his overall tied around his waist—the closest thing to pants in this place—and sported a fresh high-top fade. A familiar cartoon jingle played, and my mopping slowed as the show caught my attention.

"You down with the Inspector?" he asked.

"Hell yeah," I replied. I used to smoke weed and watch *Inspector Gadget*, a children's cartoon about a bumbling robotic cop and his nemesis, Dr. Claw.

The big guy gestured for me to sit down beside him. Leaning over conspiratorially he said, "The little girl knows what's up.

The Inspector don't know shit." We watched and laughed when Dr. Claw's pet, M.A.D. Cat, emitted a hissing little guffaw. "Here comes Chief Quimby. He's in charge," the big guy said as Gadget's boss came on the screen.

"Hey P.G.," Scraggly Beard yelled, interrupting our cartoon. "Get back on that mop!"

Jolted out of TV reverie, my new pal pulled his shoulders back, revealing his refrigerator bulk, and hollered at Scraggly Beard, "Shut the fuck up!" He looked at me and then back at Scraggly. "Ain't it your turn to mop?"

Scraggly Beard shrugged, suddenly deferential. "Mop the floor your own damn self," my new friend said. "And from here on, do P.G.'s mopping too."

"Thanks," I said. "I guess you're Chief Quimby around here," I offered. He laughed, accepting the nickname. With nothing but time, nicknames spread quickly.

"Where you from, anyway?" Chief Quimby asked.

"Canada," I said.

"Oh. That explains why you drank my milk."

Chief Quimby was local, from Seaside, California, and here on drugs and weapons charges. He was chatty, explaining who was who and how things worked. Nobody in charge of this institution ever told you what was going on—there was no orientation video or welcome package—so you came to understand the institution slowly and by osmosis. It seeped into your skin. If you were lucky, you made a friend, or found somebody to mentor you, like Chief Quimby. I listened intently as he broke down the slang and racial dynamics. "People stick to their own," he explained. Being a young, albino foreigner probably bought me a little tolerance for breaking the segregation norms.

Even drugs were racially coded, Chief Quimby explained. Crack was cheaper and more common in poor Black communities. Powder cocaine was more expensive and snorted by rich white people. Crack is not so different from powder cocaine—it's just cocaine and baking soda cooked up into crystals. Smoking rock gives you more of a rush than snorting coke, but injecting it is faster than either. Yet news coverage warned that crack was a violence-inducing plague sweeping American cities. It was a moral panic about who was using the drug, not the route of administration.

Fear of "crack babies" had spread across the continent. A now-disproved study by Dr. Ira Chasnoff suggested that babies born to women who smoked rock were much more likely to have birth defects, strokes and sudden infant death syndrome. California representative George Miller even warned that "these babies are going to overwhelm every social service delivery system that they come in contact with." Babies were seized and mothers arrested. Dr. Chasnoff's study was actually picking up on the effects of poor nutrition, lack of prenatal care and premature birth that came along with poverty and racism. The fear that the study touched off was more about race and class than chemistry.

President Ronald Reagan's Republican administration had enacted the Anti-Drug Abuse Act, which had been authored by then Democratic senator (and eventual president) Joe Biden. The law's 100:1 rule set out sentences a hundred times harsher for crack than for coke. Half a kilo of powder coke (that's real weight!) or five grams of rock (a good night for a few people) would get you the same mandatory five-year sentence. Reagan and Biden had together overcrowded my pod with poor, Black rock smokers, but there were no white, coke-snorting stock-brokers here.

Chief Quimby liked talking about food more than drugs. He had a secret barbecue rib recipe, he told me, and was shocked to learn that I was a vegetarian. He'd never met anybody who didn't eat meat. In the next breath, he asked if I would trade my sloppy joes for his vegetables, dessert and some instant coffee and tobacco. I happily agreed. That night I had a pretty decent meal, followed by coffee and a cigarette.

It felt luxurious, since I couldn't afford to buy coffee, tobacco or anything else from the commissary with the change I had in my pocket when I was arrested. We all got one cup of coffee with breakfast, but the lukewarm liquid turned grey when cream was added. Rumour had it that this beverage contained saltpetre to reduce sexual urges.

Chief Quimby was a big guy who needed way more food than the California Department of Corrections was willing to provide, so he often traded and always had big commissary orders, which broadened the options for me. I traded food with others too, scheduling my trades days in advance. The menu was the same every week, and everyone knew it by heart. Pizza Wednesdays. Fried chicken Fridays. An exchange rate emerged for these sought-after meals, but not for breakfast, which often consisted of SOS, or shit on a shingle: a scoop of greyish meat on a slice of Wonder Bread. Nobody wanted that. I swapped meat for candy, vegetables, noodles and more coffee and tobacco. I got to know more people and became a valued part of the economy.

At random, a clean piece of our uniform would be issued and the dirty ones retrieved. A guard would throw a sack into the pod and yell, "Drawers!" All twenty-seven of us would stop what we were doing, strip down and give over our underwear, waiting obediently to be issued well-worn clean pairs. Humiliation was an everyday part of life, and people held tight to whatever scraps of dignity they could. Two guys played chess with a board and pieces they'd made out of cardboard and plastic packaging from commissary items. When the pod got tossed by COs, the set was seized as contraband. After the guards were done, the players started making a new board.

When my prisoner number was finally barked over the PA, a CO escorted me to a phone-booth-sized room. My court-appointed lawyer, called a public defender, was on the other side of a thick, scratched-up Plexiglas wall. She looked down at a file, then up at me and said, "You've been charged with felony burglary under Section 459 of the California Penal Code." She looked back at the file. "And another felony, under Section 11377(a) of California's Health and Safety Code. Unlawful possession of methamphetamine or certain other narcotics." She kept talking, but I stopped hearing her. Two felonies. This was very serious. This was life-changing. In tough-on-crime, three-strikes-you're-out California, I was in deep shit.

"A felony changes everything. Employers are not going to hire you. You won't be able to get food stamps or housing vouchers." She'd obviously given this speech before. She never asked if I was guilty. It was as if I'd already been convicted.

"I'm not a US citizen," I said, but I don't think she was listening or maybe she couldn't hear me. "How long will I be here?" I said, raising my voice to be heard through the Plexiglas.

"Too soon to say," she said, packing up her briefcase. "See you in court."

"Court? When?" I shouted too late. She was already gone, off to the next little cubicle. To her, I was a number. Rushed, low-quality interactions like this were why court-appointed public defender lawyers were called "public pretenders" by everyone on my pod.

I was being digested by a bureaucracy I didn't understand. There was nobody to appeal to here. Nobody seemed to be in charge. But in our pod, there were a couple of self-professed jailhouse legal experts with many years of experience in the California penal system. Chief Quimby introduced me to the guy he always went to. We struck a deal: if he gave me some advice, I'd help him write a letter to his girlfriend. I filled him in on the details of my situation. "On the upside," he said, "this is your first serious offence. But on the downside, you got no chance of ROR (release on own recognizance) since you're from out of state." He estimated that I could be looking at two years, less a day. "Get comfortable, P.G.," said Chief Quimby.

If this was going to be my home for two years, I needed to expand my network and get to understand the place better. Walking the perimeter of the yard, a concrete room open to the sky, with a basketball hoop but no ball, I fell into conversation with other prisoners doing the same thing. I soon realized that almost all of my pod was locked up for some kind of drug-related offence. And as I heard more gossip, I found out that the same was true for guys in the pods above, beside and across from mine. They were in here for drugs too. I didn't know exactly where the prison was or even how big it was. But I learned that the pods were stacked into wings, and these wings extended into complexes, and these complexes could be found throughout the state, stretching across the vast California landscape.

This was the Game. This was the Life. And now we just had to run out the clock. All there was to do was wait. We waited for court dates, girlfriend visits and public defender consults. We waited for commissary orders, fried chicken Fridays and for *Dance Party USA* to come on at four. We waited for Inspector Gadget to solve the case. We waited for our release dates. We were always bored. In the pod, you could smoke, chat, watch TV or read one of the Louis L'Amour cowboy novels that were kicking around. I lay on my bunk and counted the ceiling tiles. I'd do anything to kill the boredom.

I'm not really the churchgoing type, but when Sunday rolled around, I jumped at any opportunity to get out of the pod. Prisoners were collected and marched to a different concrete room where we were chained together, wrist and waist, and sat on benches. Two elderly ladies led the proceedings; one did the talking, the other played a little keyboard when it was time for hymns.

"We have so much to thank Jesus for, even in a place like this. Now let's sing 'The Old Rugged Cross' . . . You know that even sinners can be saved if you repent?" When we got to "Amazing

Grace," the keyboard player encouraged us to wave our hands in time to the music. I wasn't doing it, but the hard man next to me was really into it. Since we were chained at the wrist, my lack of enthusiasm was cramping his style. "Wave yer fuckin hands," he muttered through a clenched smile. I waved my hands.

"Does anyone here feel moved to make a spiritual commitment to Christ today?" the talking lady asked. This was the altar call. Those who saw the light of the Lord were supposed to go to the front and accept Jesus. Not bloody likely, I thought. But some guy down in the front popped up, dragging the neighbours he was chained to as he tried to come forward. A CO hollered, "Sit yer ass down." No altar call today.

Boredom spawned innovation. One guy made paint by scraping magazine ads with a safety razor to create a fine powder and adding spit. Another guy made tattoo ink from cigarette ash and oil. A couple of guys fermented pruno. They collected everyone's oranges and bought sugar from the commissary. A few days later, we all got to dip our cups into a bucket that smelled like dumpster juice but gave you a good buzz.

In lower-security situations where you were allowed to order in materials for crafts, the artistry bloomed. But here, in the high-surveillance environment of my pod, constant shakedowns meant that all of this stuff would be confiscated on a regular basis, including pictures and paintings of loved ones. As with the chess players, the artisans would just start again.

My court date finally arrived, and I was shackled with other prisoners into a chain gang. A CO with a shotgun marched us onto a bus with metal grates welded over the windows. The bus took off for the courthouse—wherever that was.

We were offloaded in the courthouse basement, a dozen of us crammed into each of the courthouse's holding cells, where we waited to be taken up to the courtroom to face the judge. The cells had a bench on each wall, one toilet in the corner and no cots. The food was cold and worse than back in my pod. We waited all day. Some of us were called, but many of our appearances didn't come. At the end of the day, we were bused back to the pod, and a few days later, we were chained up and the whole process started again. Then, after a few more days, a third time. Lucky for me, Gizmo ended up in my holding cell.

Gizmo was a very little guy in his early twenties. He said he'd smoked rock since he was nine. His voice was high and he talked fast, like a cartoon character. Gizmo knew everybody and entertained the cell with hilarious stories that helped pass the time.

When he asked me what I was in for, I told him, and he said: "Don't worry. I'll tell you what to do." Gizmo lowered his voice to imitate the judge. He wagged a finger at me and said in an official tone, "Son, are you sorry?" "Yes," he answered himself, imitating me, wide-eyed and innocent. "Would you like to be released on your own recognizance?" Gizmo said, imitating the judge again. Everyone was laughing now. Then Gizmo pretended to be me again, batting his eyelashes at the judge and nodding his head, "Yessir. I'll be good. I'll be good." Now everyone was slapping their thighs and some were tearing up. "That's what you tell 'em, P.G. Tell 'em you'll be good." I laughed too. But if I got out of this, I really would try to be good.

Eventually, a CO took me, Gizmo and the rest of the cell upstairs and into the courtroom. We were lined up in three rows along the wall, chained together in our red uniforms. It was not like TV at all. There was no wood panelling. No goddess of justice, balancing her scales. No wigs and no gavel. This was a factory. In rapid succession, the court clerk called cases, prisoners stood at attention, public defenders had terse, rapid-fire exchanges with deputy district attorneys. Pleas were entered and sentences rendered. One offender sat back down, and the next number was called. The conveyor belt moved on. This was a giant machine for warehousing people—disproportionately Black and brown people. Mostly for drugs.

I was a ball of nerves by the time the court clerk called my number. I stood, commanding my knees not to shake. My charges were read out. The public defender entered a plea of "no contest" on my behalf. The judge sentenced me to time served. It was over in seconds, and the next case was called. I sat down, and another prisoner stood to be judged. I didn't know what had happened.

Gizmo elbowed me in the ribs and winked. "Time served means you are free, P.G.," he rhymed. I was going to be released in a few hours. I would have jumped for joy—had I not been chained to everyone. It had been two weeks—not two years.

That night, I said goodbye to the pod and was processed out in my socks. My boots were stored in an evidence locker at another facility. I begged the CO to let me wear my jail sandals. He relented. Released and free, I bought smokes and went to a Dairy Queen, where I drank the best cup of coffee I've ever had in my entire lifetime. A guy at one of the tables recognized my footwear and commented, "Just escaped, did ya? Right on, brother."

We Will Delete All This

Zippo and I slipped through the lobby of an old art deco apartment building at 750 O'Farrell Street in San Francisco's Tenderloin district. We climbed the stairs to the roof. Zippo was tall and skinny, like me. We both had the same slouchy gait. But I had a squint and a spiky platinum mohawk. Zippo had a shaved head and a sneer of disapproval, like some kind of art critic.

I was nineteen. I'd never done heroin before. Probably because it had a bad rep. But tonight, I didn't care. *Whatever happens, happens,* I thought.

By the light of an old pyramid skylight, Zippo cooked up our little ball of black tar. It was as thick and sticky as Athabasca bitumen. He'd done this before. I held my lighter under the spoon, and Zippo prodded the heroin with the plunger of his syringe to nudge it from solid into liquid. The smell of butane and burning spoon curled around us. I tore off a little chunk of a cigarette filter and put it in the spoon. We each drew thirty units up through that "cotton" into our own syringe. I pushed up the sleeve of my biker jacket for a tourniquet. A big vein at the inside of my left elbow jumped out to meet me, as fat as the E string on a bass guitar. It vibrated in readiness under my index finger. I took a breath and thought of the Vietnam vet who lived on Van Ness Avenue. He used to say, "Slow is smooth and smooth is fast." I repeated the phrase to myself and, in the low light, I slid the needle into my vein and pushed down the plunger.

It felt like sunshine in my veins, coming over me in warm waves. The muscles in my back and jaw relaxed. Even in the cold marine night air, I felt cozy, like a blanket had been wrapped around me. I wasn't getting wrecked. I was getting whole. I wasn't getting high. I was passing through a golden gate to a calm, protected place. Heroin was forgiveness. It was love. All the pain and tension melted away. That background howling of self-disgust was suddenly silenced. Nothing and no one could touch me here.

For years it had felt like I only had two choices: I could give up and accept that I was some kind of congenital fuck-up, flawed from birth. Or I could struggle to overcome who I was and become someone else. Now I saw a whole new path. I could just accept myself. On heroin, I didn't feel ugly. I didn't feel stupid. I didn't feel unlovable. I felt like *nothing* at all. I watched the reptile ghost boy get up and walk out into the tundra's warm midnight sun.

This was the purest kind of relief I'd ever known. *This must be what everybody else feels like all the time,* I thought. *This must be "normal."* The search was over. For me heroin wasn't self-destruction, it was salvation.

In the glow of his cigarette cherry, Zippo's scowl eased. We were like the foil soft pack of Camels in my pocket: smooth, combustible, easily crushed. Far away, cars drove empty streets and a dog barked. Somewhere out on San Francisco Bay, a ship's horn sounded a long, lonely moan. Zippo and I leaned back under the dilated night sky. Our eyelids, at half mast, let in the weak light from long-dead stars. If I let go of the tarry roof, I could fall into black forever and be gone. If I just let go.

In a deep nod, I struggled momentarily to breathe, letting out a little piggy snort that startled us both. We laughed. How long have we been here? The street was quiet now. It was somewhere between too late and too early, the wolf's tail of civil twilight. I could feel the reverie already starting to fade. But I knew I'd be back for more.

After that night on the roof, Zippo and I grew close. He was my roommate, confidant and business partner. We had each other's six. Sometimes we travelled together. We were part of a small community of teenage punks and street kids who ranged up and down the west coast. Everyone had a nickname: Jezebel, Nuk-Nuk, Knocks, Dusty, Double-D, T.J., Trash Girl, Fraggle, Zero. And—like every other city I've lived in—there was someone called Baby, someone called Animal and someone called Mama Bear.

We were living through the supposed "end of history." Capitalism had beaten the Soviets. All the important battles were over. And we were supposed to be happy about it all. It was the era between 1960s Summer of Love San Francisco and the tech-bro dystopia that characterized the city in the 2000s. In this interregnum, hella morbid symptoms appeared: Polk Street hustlers, black tar heroin and East Bay punk rock. It was Kerouac's end-of-land sadness. California noir.

In other cities, you could couch surf. But here, everyone's sofa had a waiting list. So Zippo and I squatted in a vacant house with a sagging, out-of-tune piano. We squatted in an old abandoned warehouse. We camped upstairs in a half-demolished record store, wading through drifts of vinyl on the first floor. Wherever we stayed, Zippo and I slept in the same room, for camaraderie and safety. Every night, we'd roll out the sleeping bags, put on our Joy Division tape, and fall asleep to Ian Curtis's bleak, reverb-soaked lullabies. The cops always kicked us out eventually. One time they surrounded our building. Over a megaphone, they ordered us to exit quietly or they'd send in a K9 unit to flush us out.

When I wasn't squatting with Zippo, I stayed at Star's. She was a dancer. Her every movement was graceful—even when she was counting change. Star worked at the Market Street Cinema, a grand old movie house turned strip club, known to those who worked there as the Market Street Enema. Four or five nights a week, Star took the stage, put down a bed sheet and danced a set of three songs—maybe Ministry, the Cure and Sisters of Mercy. Then she'd go into the audience and lap dance for tips. She asked me to help choose songs but I never went to see her dance. I didn't want it to change how she saw me.

At around two a.m., I'd pick Star up at the Cinema's side door. We'd walk back to her little room in a cheap hotel next to the bus station. Star would unsnap the body suit she was required to wear and backflip across the floor to retrieve a glass of water. She didn't care if I did dope, as long as I wasn't nodding out when we were together.

Most weekends, I volunteered at Gilman Street, an all-ages club that put on the best gigs: Jawbreaker, Neurosis, J Church, Blatz. Every inch was covered in graffiti and handbills. It was run by a collective of kids who played in the bands. Volunteers like me could sleep on the floor at the end of the night. Rules were written by the door: no racism, no sexism, no violence—but also no drugs. I had to keep my habit a secret here.

With Zippo's help, I learned San Francisco's public transit system—a homicide detective's yarn diagram of interconnecting train lines and stations, tying together all our squats, friends' flats, coffee spots, dealers and petty scams. My bad eyesight made it hard to visualize a map. Instead, I learned the *story* of how to get somewhere. In this case, told in Zippo's twangy Montana accent.

A year had passed since I first did heroin, and now I had a habit. It had come on cunningly, bit by bit. But now there was no denying it: I was wired. Evening was coming by the time Zippo and I dragged ourselves to the Tenderloin. The dirty winter fog off San Francisco Bay had worked its way under my hoodie and into my lungs. A cold, stalactite sweat slithered down my spine. I was restless, anxious and sniffly. I was feeling the early symptoms of withdrawal. Dopesickness felt like divine justice—God's punishment for daring to feel good. I should've seen it coming.

Zippo was jonesing too. We squabbled for ten minutes about what to do next, that antsy, dopesick feeling building up RPMs. The clock was running and worse symptoms were coming.

We hurried past strip clubs, liquor stores, historic gay bars, rooming houses and pawn shops. The frenetic business of the day was being coughed onto the sidewalks. Everyone took a deep breath. And the rain started.

We were wet and miserable by the time we reached Glide Church. This place put on a good breakfast at eight a.m. But what I really loved was the music. When the congregation sang "Let It Shine" or "There Is Hope," their voices broke into exquisite harmonies, accompanied by a tight rhythm section, clapping hands and a brass ensemble. It didn't sound anything like the music I'd heard in white churches.

"Rollers," Zippo warned, just barely glancing over his shoulder at the police car creeping down Larkin Street. The cops had been on a tear, doing block-by-block sweeps, writing tickets for loitering, drinking, panhandling and "camping." We had collected a bunch of tickets.

At that time, HIV was spreading fast. It was highly stigmatized, and treatment was in its infancy. Needle distribution was illegal in most places, and if the cops caught you with a syringe, they'd confiscate it. I kept mine hidden in my boot. AIDS activists sometimes smuggled new rigs around the city in an empty baby carriage. They ran an illegal guerilla needle exchange at Civic Center. That's where I got a brand new syringe, still in its packaging. But that had been a few weeks ago. Since then, my rig had gotten dull, so I sharpened it on a matchbook striker. It still wasn't very sharp. The numbers on the barrel were fading, and the plunger wasn't running smooth anymore.

If you weren't lucky enough to get a rig from the activists, you might have to buy a used one from someone on the street, knowing it was probably contaminated. Sometimes, Zippo and I had to share one needle. Whoever went first would rinse the outfit with bleach and water before passing it to the other. In those days, we didn't know that the virus could also survive on our spoons and in our cottons. Since a bit of dope always remained in a cotton after you used it, they were shared among drug users. Cottons were little units of currency.

Zippo and I took up our usual spot on the corner of Polk and O'Farrell. Cars sizzled past on the wet pavement. Kitty-corner from us, Ponyboy was perched against a wall—shirtless as usual—smoking with little flourishes like he was in a movie from the 1940s. Pony was a stimulant-fuelled dynamo, a veteran hustler. He was nicknamed for his ponytail—which he constantly set loose and retied—not for the character from *The Outsiders*. Speed helped Pony stay alert, keep moving and sparkle through long nights and dreary dates. Commenting on how young I looked, Pony quipped: "Silly rabbit, kids are for tricks."

Zippo did sex work from time to time when he was dopesick. But he didn't do it proudly or defiantly, like Pony. For Zippo, every date was a final exception, brought on by dire circumstances. Those dates were never mentioned again. I always tried to get dope money in other ways. I'd sell items I found in our squat or go to Fisherman's Wharf and charge wide-eyed Midwestern tourists a few bucks to pose for pictures with a punk rocker. I had slept with people for drugs before, but I never thought of *that* as sex work. Now—dopesick and broke—I didn't care about such distinctions.

A middle-aged man walked up and caught Zippo's eye. They exchanged a few words that I couldn't make out, but I could tell they already knew each other. Eventually, Zippo and the man turned to look at me. "Come on," Zippo said. "This is Steve. He wants you too." As the three of us walked off together, I took a better look at Steve. He was a lot older than me and he looked straight, like the kind of guy who has a wife and kids back home. Zippo whispered to me that he'd been with this guy before, but that he wasn't a regular.

Steve was oozing with some kind of hunger. He tried to cover it over with nonchalance, but it wasn't working. He ushered us into his cheap hotel room like a maître d'. We sat at a Formica kitchen table and he passed us each a can of Colt 45. I nursed the drink, but it squirmed in my guts like an eel. I wondered if I was going to puke in front of our new employer.

Zippo refused to put people at ease with banter out of principle, preferring to keep them guessing and on edge. So I handled the perfunctory small talk. "Sure is raining a lot," I said.

"Sure is," Steve agreed, uninterested but relieved to be in some kind of conversation. "Those beers are gonna be deducted from your payment, y'know?" he joked. Nobody laughed.

Zippo pushed back from the table, showing his impatience by scraping his chair. With the same resigned efficiency as jail intake, we removed our boots and jackets. I noticed that the left knee of my jeans was flecked with little dots of blood and bleach. I could smell chemical illness coming off our bodies. Somewhere, water dripped—from a gutter or a tap—in a quick, anxiety-making tempo. Zippo's ribs showed through his back. I glanced down at my own pale skin, knowing I looked the same.

I pulled out the little zip-lock HIV/AIDS prevention kit I'd got from Larkin Street Youth Services. I fished past the bleach and water and pulled out a couple of bright yellow condoms, passing one to Zippo. We each rolled them on. I was lucky to still have the condoms—because cops were confiscating them off suspected hustlers.

"Like a marble statue," Steve breathed, looking at me in the fluorescent light from the little kitchenette. I tried not to grimace at the comment. I knew this kind of guy. He probably thought getting with an albino was an exotic accomplishment. He wanted to face me, to gaze at me.

On the bed, I positioned myself in front, shifting my hips up toward Steve's head. I felt a little guilty that I was getting the easier job. I tried to make my movements look unrushed as Zippo moved behind him. The malt liquor was sloshing inside me like bilge water. I was struggling to keep it down and my dick up. There was a fine balance to maintain. I wanted to mentally check out and not think about what I was doing. But I also had to be there physically. I remembered some wisdom Ponyboy had shared with me: "Picture some girl you've been with," he said. So, I tried to imagine Star, the dancer. But instead, my mind looped back to Victoria.

I was ten years old. Victoria was in her thirties. My parents hired her to watch me and my sister while they were at work. Victoria would take me out on "coffee dates," leaning in close and conspiratorial. Her polished nails tapped the glass tabletop to punctuate each syllable. "A good man is hard to find." Click, click, click. She gestured to me with her white ceramic mug and arched an eyebrow, giving me her total attention. I felt my heart flutter like a little chickadee in my chest. Was I the "good man" she was looking for?

Walking in the rain, we got soaked to the skin. "You're cold," Victoria said, with motherly concern. "Let's have a shower to warm up." When I hesitated, she led my little sister in, singing

"Turkey in the Straw" to embarrass me into the tub. Victoria said we were star-crossed lovers, like in *The Owl and the Pussycat*, a 1970s film we watched late one night on TV. It was about a failed writer and a sex worker. A moustache, she told me, is very attractive on a man. But I couldn't grow a moustache yet.

At the car wash, I sat in the passenger seat of her silver hatchback. Riding up front—like an adult. We sang along to Leo Sayer on the AM radio. The water and brushes beat on the roof. The soap on the windows made a private cave for us. We harmonized on the woah-woes and yay-yays of the chorus. The menthol smell of her Noxzema filled the small car.

"When you're older, we'll meet under the Eiffel Tower," she said dreamily as water ran down the windows. "I'll put aside a bottle of wine for us, until it's properly aged." *How old is "properly aged"?* I wondered. I imagined us grown-up and sophisticated, clinking long-stemmed glasses. The Eiffel Tower was tall enough to jump off. I could make her watch my body splatter on the pavement.

Victoria was mercurial, quick to anger for reasons I could never decrypt. She screamed and slapped me. My skin burned where her hand hit my face. She was jealous of a girl named Bronwyn in my grade six class. With a sneer, Victoria would mispronounce her name on purpose: "Blod-win." She was jealous of the affection I had for our small black cat, Shadow. She poisoned the little creature. It took all day for her to die.

Walking up the basement stairs, I saw Victoria at the top. She held open her long white coat, showing she had nothing underneath. The curve of hips and waist were outlined in the fluorescent light from the kitchen. I stopped in the middle.

I didn't want to go up, but I couldn't retreat. I was stuck. I sat there in my blue pyjamas. My knee jumped like a sewing machine. I turned away, my face hot and tingling. I pulled at the peeling edge of the linoleum on the step, a tangle of dark hair hovering above me. "There's nothing to be embarrassed about," she reassured, in a sex-ed teacher's sensible tone, coaxing me up the stairs. "It's natural."

A few nights later, I woke my parents. "Can't this wait until morning?" my dad asked sleepily into their dark bedroom. They were both career people who had to get up for work in a few hours.

"You can't leave us alone with Victoria," I said, my resolve already starting to melt. I felt queasy, like I was about to confess something incriminating.

"What's going on?" Dad asked. I opened my mouth to explain but I didn't have the words. Maybe they wouldn't believe me. Maybe this was my fault. Maybe they'd be disgusted. A couple of beats of silence followed. The room froze up. I froze up. There was no reaction. This did not compute. My words hung in the air for long, empty seconds, until they fell to the floor. Deleted. I said nothing more.

Looking back, I don't know if my parents were even fully awake. If I had been able to find the words, I think they would've done something. But that moment was a microscopic virus that multiplied and mutated, infecting the future. My relationship with them would never be the same. Something was ending between us.

Sleepless, back in the basement, with battery-acid taste in my mouth, I listened for footfalls on the stairs. I held my breath. I could hear the background hum of my own brain. I didn't want to hear her footsteps, but I also missed them. I rocked myself in my Pac-Man sheets, with four little colourful, pixelated ghosts—Inky, Blinky, Pinky and Clyde—fleeing from the all-consuming mouth.

Victoria talked about how real monsters were out there. Like the serial child killer Clifford Robert Olson. But she called herself "the devil you know." I was lucky, Victoria said. Some of the kids at school had no one to look after them while their parents worked. She was the only one who would take care of me. She said, "Vaginas are all neat and tucked away. Not like a man"—a twinge of disgust changing the sound of her words—"all dangling out there, messy." She meant me. I was messy and ugly. She called my sister "the little gooseberry"—a third wheel, an unwanted extra person on a date. A witness.

Through Victoria's eyes, I came into focus, not a part of anything, but apart from everything. A skinny kid with a bowl cut and Coke-bottle glasses. Spare parts. A pale cave creature, evolved to live alone in the dark. Repulsive to everyone—except her. She was enthralled. She drew close. She started listening to the same music as me. She cut her hair short and bleached it to look like mine.

I threw out the stuffed Garfield toy my aunt Rose had given me. I wasn't a baby anymore. Victoria made me older. I drove eight self-tapping Robertson screws into the frame of my bedroom door, securing a single hinge hasp lock. By consensus of all the men in my family, Robertson was best. It doesn't strip. I leaned my skinny, ninety-pound body into the screwdriver. With every clockwise rotation, I twisted away from my parents. They could never know this filthy, broken part of me. Or the part that lived only to numb it all out. I drove another screw into the door. *Righty-tighty. Nighty-nighty.*

I shook off the memory of Victoria and found Steve staring at me. I could feel my own eyes shake like a glitching robot, looking at nothing. Zippo knew the trick was almost done and adjusted his tempo. Zippo caught my eye and held my gaze for a beat. I looked back at him. Zippo subtly shook his head from side to side. I knew exactly what he meant. He meant: *We will delete all this.*

Steve finished, and the mood switched in an instant. He stood up and began pacing. I wondered what was going on. Was he going to rip us off? Zippo noticed too. The possibility of violence crackled in the air. But wait, he wasn't being shady, just shameful. He wanted something forbidden, he got it, and this was just its bitter aftertaste.

Steve paid us, and we bolted with unlaced boots and unzipped jeans. The rain had stopped. On the quickmarch down Polk Street to score, we paid each other the tender respect of silence, entering an unspoken pact of forgetting. Zippo spat. I jammed my hand down my jeans, pulled off the forgotten yellow condom and threw it in the gutter. Zippo and I got our dope and went back to the roof at 750 O'Farrell Street to fix.

Hours later, we came down and went into a corner store for a soda. I was still nodding hard, in front of the cooler. I slumped down onto the floor, unable to choose a pop. The guy behind the till got cranky, so Zippo walked me outside into the cold IOU of dawn. "Let's go home and put on the Joy Division tape," he said.

PART 2
GETTING
DOPESICK

Don't Fuck It Up

'd been to plenty of punk shows, but this was my first time performing at one. I was the singer in a band I'd just formed with three other friends called Lumpin Proletariat. We had a three-chord anti-fascist song called "Follow Your Leader." The lyrics encouraged local far-right thugs to follow Hitler into the dustbin of history. The audience, a couple dozen people in an Ottawa basement, were all people we knew. They cheered and made fun of us during our half-hour set.

We struck our last chord to a smattering of applause, then the drummer and I snuck off into the snowy night, looking for morphine. We'd heard a woman just up the street had some.

We were floating by the time we got back to the venue. But— to our surprise—we found that no one was in the basement anymore; everyone was arguing out on the street. A group of Nazi skinheads from the Heritage Front were there. They'd heard about our lyrics and wanted to do something about it. The basement was already trashed. Now the street was a tense standoff.

I squinted, trying to figure out where the threats might come from. Was anyone holding a bottle? Was anyone holding a knife? I stood up straight. The Nazis didn't know that I was blind, but they could see that I was tall. And over the years I'd found I could often avoid violence simply by looking like I would fight back. I had become pretty good at acting totally unafraid.

In the chaos, a guy with long hair approached me. He appeared to be in his mid-twenties—just a few years older than me. He hadn't been at the show, so I figured he must have walked up on the street. Right away I was struck by how nonchalant he seemed. He had an easygoing, casual stance—he didn't seem fazed by the violence that was about to break out. But I could tell he was ready to jump in, if the need arose.

"What's going on here?" he asked me.

"Punks against Nazis," I said.

"Nazis?" he mumbled, balling up his fists.

A siren sounded and people fled down the side streets. Suddenly the world was still again.

"What's your name?" I asked.

"Jeff," he replied. "Jeff Louden."

Jeff and I stood around in the snowy street for a while, chatting aimlessly. He seemed like an interesting guy. I asked him where he lived and was surprised to learn he was staying in a rooming house kitty-corner to my place.

The next day I walked across the street and knocked on Jeff's door. He invited me in and we climbed the stairs to his room, which was decked out with the same used or dumpster-dived furniture as my place. Beside his hot plate was a little television set.

"Nice TV," I said, trying to make small talk.

"It's black-and-white," Jeff responded. "And it only gets two channels." Jeff gestured to the rabbit-ears antenna. "I'll trade it for a case of beer."

"Sure," I said.

That afternoon, Jeff and I drank the beer together while watching reruns of *Gunsmoke* and *North of 60*. I eventually got up to go, deciding to leave the TV at his place. After all, I drank plenty of his beer.

"Don't forget the tube," Jeff called after me.

"What are you gonna watch then?" I asked.

"There's plenty more where that came from," Jeff said, insisting I take it. "Something'll fall off the back of a truck."

Before long, Jeff and I were hanging out, drinking and watching TV together nearly every night. He came to watch my band rehearse. We even exchanged house keys. I learned that Jeff was Anishinaabe, born on the Curve Lake First Nation reserve in southern Ontario. He told me he didn't remember much about his mother or community because he'd been adopted by a white family in Toronto. Eventually that family gave Jeff up, and he bounced around the foster system, a place rampant with racism, neglect and abuse. Jeff was only nine when he entered the system. At that age, I was going to summer camp, swimming lessons, canoe trips and a family vacation to Disneyland. My life couldn't have been more different.

Jeff told me that—like me—he'd been bullied as a kid. He had a small birthmark on the end of his nose—just large enough that the other kids couldn't resist tormenting him. All these years later, I could tell Jeff was still self-conscious about it. But I couldn't see it at all. I found it difficult enough to differentiate his nose from the rest of his face. From my point of view, I told Jeff, there was nothing wrong with his nose at all. Later, when he had the birthmark removed, I didn't even notice.

After foster care, Jeff did time in various institutions for juvenile offenders. And, later, in jails and prisons. Colonial violence had marked every phase of his life, leaving him with what I could only imagine were serious psychological scars. Jeff soothed his pain with heroin, just like me. But he'd found the solution a lot earlier than I did.

"I was nine," Jeff told me. "It was love at first fix."

That summer Jeff and I worked our way through a formulary of pharmaceuticals. I could feel the habit I'd had in San Francisco creeping back, but I stopped short of getting totally wired. Pills were very common in Ottawa. It was easy to find prescription opioids, stimulants, hypnotics, benzodiazepines and barbiturates. Sometimes we got them prescribed to us by actual doctors. We crushed, cooked and injected them. We both liked the grey morphine pills, and sometimes we shot Ts & Rs (Talwin and Ritalin), a painkiller-and-stimulant combination known as the poor man's speedball. We did Vicodin, Oxy, Percocet, clonidine, Rivotril, phenobarbital and fentanyl. Heroin was rare. But when we could track some down, it was our drug of choice.

Jeff was only four years older than me, but he'd been in the life much longer. Sometimes I felt like his understudy. He showed me cooking tricks, techniques and recipes he'd learned in prison. He also taught me to better defend myself. "It's not really so much about eyesight," he said. "It's about listening to your gut." I tried to see the street the way he did. How to talk someone down. How to clock potential threats. Jeff said you don't need to worry so much about the guy running his mouth with menace and bravado. It's the quiet guys you've got to keep an eye on. I tried to mimic Jeff's impassive toughness. But no one could do it like him.

Jeff had a quick retort for everything. He would defuse tension and deflect interest with sharp one-liners, keeping everyone at arm's length. He was a loner, but over time, I caught glimpses of Jeff's gentler side. He loved animals and told me he wrote poetry. I asked if I could read some, but Jeff was too shy to show me. I didn't let it go, and eventually—after weeks of pestering—he tossed me his notebook. Jeff told me to read it later, by myself. At home, I read the poems. Some were dark. He wrote about the Grim Reaper, about violence, death and survival. His lines could have been metal lyrics.

Before long, Jeff and I were best friends.

One Monday, I woke up to the smell of brewing coffee. I found Jeff in my kitchen, pouring us both a cup. I didn't recognize the pair of oxblood-red Doc Martens sitting by the door, snow melting off them.

"New boots?" I asked.

"New to you," Jeff replied. He explained that on the way over he'd spotted a Nazi skinhead casing my place. Jeff described the guy, and I said it sounded like a Heritage Front member. One of them had threatened to Molotov my apartment with his buddies. I wasn't sure how serious they were, but I was worried. "I dummied the guy and took his boots," Jeff shrugged. He always answered in short sentences—as if what he was saying was obvious. As if knocking someone out was barely worth a mention. "I left him in the snowbank to walk home in socks. I think they're your size."

———

In 1993, after a North American tour with the band, I moved back to British Columbia. Jeff had moved there a few months earlier. The drug scene in Vancouver couldn't have been more different. Heroin had been pretty hard to find in Ottawa. But in Vancouver, "China White" heroin was stronger than anything the city had seen before, and it was easy to find in the blocks around Main and Hastings. The scandalized press called the area an "open-air drug market." Overdoses were spiking—that year, there were a record 354 overdose deaths in BC. Ambulances were racing back and forth to prone bodies on the sidewalk. But to us, the high potency wasn't as much a risk as a selling point. Crack had also arrived in Vancouver. We would shoot speedballs—heroin and coke together in the same syringe. The shit was good.

Ever since I first did dope on that rooftop in San Francisco and felt it drain me of all my shame and self-hate, I couldn't stay away. I used whenever I had the money. After a year or so in Vancouver, I was wired again—using every day or dopesick if I didn't. There was no middle ground. Soon I had a gram-a-day habit, and those beautiful moments of euphoria had become less frequent. More often, I was doing dope just to relieve dopesickness. Heroin was once my salvation. But now I was just trying not to feel ill.

I'd always heard about "lazy junkies." But nothing could be further from the truth. When you're wired, the misery of dope-sickness is always just around the corner. And the only thing that can keep it at bay is money. And so we had to hustle. But there was still never enough cash.

Then one day Jeff was gone. At first I had no idea what happened—he had just disappeared. But a week later, the phone rang. I picked up and a robot voice said, "You are receiving a call from an inmate at the Vancouver Island Regional Correctional Centre." It was Jeff. He said he'd been arrested on some old warrants and was locked up in Wilkinson Road, a maximum-security facility that looked like a medieval castle.

Politicians often claim they'll get drugs off the streets, but the truth is they can't even keep them out of the jails. I was worried that Jeff was struggling with withdrawal, but he assured me that things were okay. We didn't talk about it on the phone, but I remembered that Jeff knew how to distill alcohol and sell it to other prisoners for dope money. Jeff also knew how to make a syringe out of a Bic pen and a piece of sneaker rubber.

I sent Jeff commissary money and a letter with a cartoon. The first panel showed me riding a gigantic rig full of dope. I was hurtling through the sky, waving a cowboy hat, like Slim Pickens in *Dr. Strangelove*. In the second panel, the rig and I smashed through the jail walls, injecting Jeff with a big load of dope. In the third panel, Jeff and I rode off on the needle, reunited and free.

Jeff's letter back was written in block letters—neat and big enough for me to easily read. He said he loved the cartoon, but the warden had confiscated it as seditious. Then he got serious.

Garth, I didn't want to fuck your life up for you. I figure if you want that path, you're better at your own speed. The speed I travel at is too fast for anyone. And now I must pay, I guess. The rabbit is once again locked in a cage. Your friend, Jeff.

I wanted to tell Jeff that he was wrong. That he wasn't going too fast for me. That we were on the same page. But deep down I knew he was right. Although he would never admit it, the Canadian state had inflicted a deep wound in Jeff. And he was compelled to anaesthetize it with as much dope as possible. Jeff knew who he was, and he wasn't apologizing for it.

I had cobbled together an undergraduate degree in sociology with courses taken at colleges and universities in Ottawa, Quebec City and Victoria. And I knew that I had a knack for writing. But I also knew that if I didn't make a big change soon, I'd be fucked.

I considered my options and decided to apply to graduate school at the London School of Economics. LSE is the place where sociology was supposedly invented, and the campus had a strong leftist history. It was also the kind of place where heads of state studied—clearly, way out of my league, I thought, but worth a shot. When a letter from the school finally arrived, I assumed it would say, "Thank you, but you aren't what we're looking for." I had to read it twice before I understood that it was a letter of acceptance.

I started making preparations. I gave notice to my landlord and applied for a passport, bursaries and student loans. A few days before my departure, my mom, dad, sister, aunt, uncle and I went out for dinner to celebrate and say goodbye. I picked at my fries. I had a lot of dope on board, so I couldn't eat much. I wondered if my mom noticed I wasn't eating. My aunt and uncle gave me a card wishing me well, with a red lai see lucky-money envelope inside. Dad raised his glass to make a toast. He said he was proud of me.

As soon as I touched down in London, I planned to kick dope forever. I'd try the geographic cure. I opened my notebook to write out a plan. I calculated how much dope I would need to last me the flight to London, plus a few hours to get to my room, check out the neighbourhood, buy some groceries and go for a pint before the withdrawal symptoms set in. I'd bring a couple of books to get a jump on the course readings while I was sick. I'd bring an old prescription bottle of clonazepam, just in case, but I was pretty sure I could do this cold turkey. I'd been through it before, and besides, I wouldn't be around any dope in London. I didn't even know what the British called it. A new city would give me a shot at becoming a new person.

As I finished writing out my detox plan, the phone rang. It was Jeff again. He tried not to call too often because it was not cheap. But I was glad he did today. I told Jeff I'd been accepted to LSE and that I was moving to London. He told me he was proud of me. It was bittersweet. We both knew we wouldn't see each other again for years—maybe forever. The line clicked and hummed in our awkward silence. Jeff broke the tension by teasing me about becoming a tea-slurping crumpet-muncher. I laughed sadly, feeling like a traitor. How could I go on this exciting adventure while Jeff languished in jail? I felt like we were heading in opposite directions, and I worried our friendship would never be the same—especially after I quit dope. Jeff could always tell what I was feeling. "Worry about your own self," he snapped at me, "and don't fuck it up." I promised I'd do my best.

The Shipping Forecast

At Vancouver International Airport, I slid into a bathroom stall and locked the door. I laid out a piece of toilet paper on the metal dispenser and set out my rig, lighter, cotton, water, spoon and my last flap of dope. I fake-coughed to cover the flick of my lighter and did my last hit ever before beginning my new life. It smoothly attenuated the roar of boarding announcements, hand dryers and flushing toilets.

I slept most of the way across. Somewhere over the sea off Baffin Island, I woke up to find a rectangle of cold pasta on the table tray in front of me. I didn't know how it got there, but I knew I wouldn't be touching the stuff. Hours later the food was gone and the table tray was up. Meridians of longitude clicked by, and I felt okay. So far, everything was going to plan.

We landed at Gatwick Airport, and the plane took ages to unload. I started becoming conscious of time. I waited in the customs and immigration line for an hour, then answered another twenty minutes of questions from an immigration officer. The first shivers of dopesickness were hitting me. I could feel the handle of my guitar case getting heavy. "Welcome to the United Kingdom," the immigration officer finally said, noticing the queue forming behind me. He stamped my passport and waved me on. I waited for the train into London. Everything was taking much longer than I had calculated.

By the time I got to my Central London student room, a gale-force storm was raging in my stomach. The constipation of prolonged opioid use was ending violently, and I was in full-blown withdrawal. I threw my bags on the ground and rushed to the bathroom. Sitting on the toilet, I let my head loll in the sink beside me. Dark liquid shot from both ends and into Sir Bazalgette's sewers until there was nothing left.

Shaking, I crawled to the bed and lay there sweating. I was tired but restless and anxious. I was expecting all this, it was all part of the plan, but that didn't make it feel any better. Desperate for distraction, I dug out my radio, thumbing the dial through unfamiliar stations until I landed on an authoritative British accent. "And now the shipping forecast from the Met Office. Low England 1005 expected FitzRoy 1010 by midnight Saturday. Low. Biscay, Dogger, Fisher, German Bight 1004 slow moving and falling."

It was a mysterious maritime poem of place names, wind, weather, sea states and visibility. The broadcast repeated every six hours as my symptoms got worse and worse. I couldn't hold down food or water. Meteorological measurements and withdrawal symptoms blurred together.

Low Biscay losing its identity. Pulse rising slowly. Viking, North Utsire, South Utsire, Restless seas. Doom increasing. Gale force vomit warning, Visibility descending. Nerves occasionally poor. Forties, Cromarty, Forth, Fever increasing. Tyne, Dogger, Northeasterly chills. Expect repeated shakes.

Fisher, German Bight, Humber, Trafalgar, Finisterre, Heart
pounding. Sole, Lundy, Fastnet, Cramps, Shannon, Rockall,
Malin, Insomnia Automatic. Trembling Hebrides, Bailey, Fair
Isle fucked up, Southeast Iceland suicidal ideation.

I lay on one side for a few seconds, but it became intolerable so I thrashed onto the other side. Then back again. I rocked back and forth—the old rhythmic movement re-emerging. The damp sheet twisted around me, mummifying me. My legs involuntarily kicked out a panicky SOS in Morse code. The nuclear forces holding all my atoms together seemed to be weakening. I felt like I was coming apart.

Dope is like floating in space, free from the pull of gravity and the noise of the world. But kicking is re-entry without a heat shield—you break apart in the atmosphere like a malfunctioning satellite. Dragged down. Burnt up.

After three days, there was still no let-up. I had nothing left to vomit. I had no energy to shiver or thrash around. The slightest move hurt, so I just lay still, staring up at the ceiling. It was the same colour as London's wet skies. I didn't know what day it was or when classes were supposed to start. My plan was out the window. The dope was draining out of each cell in my body.

The room smelled like chemical illness—like a sick robot. This was the worst yet. Each time I had tried to kick, the symptoms had been more severe than the last. The first few times, back in California, I didn't really know what to expect. But now my brain knew what was coming, and that made it worse. They call it the Kindling Effect, and I was ablaze with illness.

I swallowed a handful of clonazepam, the pills I had hoped to save for emergencies. Immediately, I ran to the sink and threw them up. I didn't have enough to waste, so I washed them off and shoved the puked pills up my ass. If you can't hold anything down, "suitcasing" is the only option. The stomach acid on the pills stung, but I didn't care.

My plan to get clean seemed ridiculous now. I was skinny and weak. I could barely lift my head off the floor. The radio jabbered away about people and places I'd never heard of. I knew nothing about this country. I had moved across the world, but I was never going to be well enough to crawl out of this little room. If by some miracle I managed to, how could I ever walk into the London School of Economics? They'd call security. All the shame and self-hate came flooding back in. I was a kid in elementary school. The ten-year-old on the basement stairs with Victoria looming at the top. I was a ghost in my own life again.

I felt sure I was going to die. Then I wanted to. I found myself in the toilet with a serrated knife in the sink. Did I unconsciously bring it in here? I felt the need to cut a small hole, a hatch to vent all the sickness out of me. But I couldn't imagine tearing into my flesh with the ugly serrations. I dropped the knife and walked back to bed. It was the most I'd moved since I got here.

The BBC was playing a slow waltz called "Sailing By." It came on before every shipping forecast. I tried to figure out how long it had been—almost a week? I was ravenously hungry. I ate some dry noodles. My body wasn't trying to kill me anymore. But now I couldn't sleep. I paced the room in a fugue state of regret and doom, boredom and self-hate. Then I left the building.

The fever world of the tangled sheets bled into the waking world of twisting streets, as I stumbled through London's snarled chaos of roads and alleys, past newspaper hawkers, old churches and the towering cylindrical metal frames of disused gasometers, glinting skeletal against the dark sky. I walked down to the Thames. It glared back, stinking, shipless and black as bitumen. The city smelled like ancient river and leaded gasoline. It was damp, but not the decaying-rainforest damp of Vancouver. London's damp was industrial. Centuries of steam and soot from Victorian factories stained the old stone walls. The city and the sky were the colour of smoke.

Bloomsbury Café was the only thing open. I sat down on a red vinyl banquette. A couple of cabbies were drinking tea and reading the paper. I ordered a full English breakfast and ate half of it. As the grease congealed on my abandoned sausages, I tried to remember why I came here and piece back together my vision of the new future I had dreamed of.

But the past was reflected back at me in the chrome napkin dispenser. It found me here. It didn't matter if I was in Yellow-knife, San Francisco or in a submarine on the bottom of Scapa Flow. You can't hide from yourself. The ghost crawled back inside. Horrible reptilian slimy feet on my skin. Swimming in my sick bloodstream. He picked up where we left off. The geographic cure is bullshit. I needed dope.

I only knew one other person in London, and I was pretty sure he'd have what I needed. I had met Sunny in Vancouver a few years earlier. We'd done dope together once or twice, and I figured he'd know where to score here. I didn't bother trying to learn the transit system. I just threw myself into it, down a long clanking escalator, through the city's layers. London was an old city, built over top of even older cities. Roman cities. I breathed in the blackdamp.

The London Underground was a creature with its own wheezy pneumatic respiration, blowing and sucking through serpentine tubes. Its circulatory system of rust had no liver. It felt as sick as me. I was just another bacterium, drifting in its bloodstream. The driver called the stations through a crackly Tannoy PA: King's Cross. Caledonian Road. My blood was screaming like a boiling kettle. Holloway Road. Arsenal. Finsbury Park . . . Another strange poem of strange places.

Finally, Manor House. Up and out in the air again. There are no straight streets in London. They change the name every couple of blocks. I navigated Hackney by narcotic dead reckoning. In new places, I just got a feeling of where to go. I tried to straighten up and walk normally. I hated looking like a drug spider. But I was the only one who cared.

Sunny saw me in the door of his squat and immediately recognized my need. I didn't have to wait. He gave me what he had and let me fix right there in his front hall. It was an incredible relief. I felt normal again. All that suffering wasn't for nothing. This was a one-time thing.

Sunny was bald, in his thirties and had a tattoo of a donkey with a giant penis. He was known as Sunshine or Sunny-boy because of his dour disposition. He simultaneously rejected and embodied Englishness. An old-school anarchist traveller, he'd squatted for ages and fought on picket lines and in the Poll Tax Riot. But like my grandfather, he was very particular about how he made his tea ("You must hot the pot"), and he watched classic British TV shows every day—*Coronation Street* and *EastEnders*. He insisted on absolute silence when *Antiques Roadshow* came on.

I was used to Mexican black tar or Vancouver's China White heroin, but Sunny's "gear" was from Afghanistan. The voltage was different in London, and cars drove on the other side of the street; why not the heroin too? In Vancouver, the white powder had been so pure you needed only to add water; cooking was optional. But this brown heroin was a little rough. It was less water-soluble. It needed help. Sunny gave me citric powder to cook it down with. "It's the shit they use for getting limescale off the kettle," he said. This brown had less kick but more creep; smooth and plenty of legs. I felt well for the first time since crossing the Atlantic.

I slid down the wall and sat on the floor, exhaling deeply, and the old ghosts and creeping doubts suddenly fell silent. The shipping forecast now predicted a calm North Sea. It was to be smooth sailing. I was never going to be able to stay white-knuckle clean. Heroin was the only thing that kept me afloat. Sunny looked down at me sitting on his hallway floor and judged me ready for a conversation.

"So, Garth, what the fuck are you doing in London? Never mind. Tell me on the way. That was the last of the gear." Since I'd helped Sunny finish off his dope, we needed to get more. We caught a red Routemaster double-decker bus and got off within spitting distance of Wessex Studios, where the Clash recorded *London Calling*. We cut across Clissold Park, our pace quickening. At the intersection of Clissold Road and Stoke Newington Church Street stood a red brick housing scheme with a rounded front. We walked through an outdoor hallway and up the stairs to an abandoned flat that locals used as a shooting gallery. Inside, there was an old couch and a couple of chairs. It was dark, except for a few candles and the watery light of a street lamp oozing through the smeared kitchen window.

Four other people were already waiting. Sunny nodded at them. "When's Skinny getting here?" he asked. A guy in the corner shrugged. Everyone was waiting for dope, and idle small talk was the only thing to do. Two guys were talking about football. A girl in the corner with growing-out black-dyed hair sighed and said—to no one in particular—"Fuck me, wish I could just pop down the chemist and not spend ages waiting on Skin." There were mumbles of resigned agreement. This was apparently a point of tired consensus. I asked what she meant. She explained that her mom's friend had been prescribed heroin for years, so she didn't have to spend all her time and money at places like Skinny's shooting gallery.

It was called the "British System," she explained. In the 1920s, British doctors started prescribing diacetylmorphine (heroin) to people with a dope habit. Heroin was dispensed at a pharmacy courtesy of the British National Health Service. Later research showed that prescribed heroin reduced HIV transmission among patients, allowed people to stabilize their lives and eliminated the need for crime to pay for dope on the street.

While the rest of the world was waging a war on drugs, the Brits were doing something totally different. It sounded too good to be true—like an urban legend. *Junkies are always talking shit,* I thought. And if they simply gave heroin away here, why was everyone waiting for Skinny in this chilly shooting gallery?

What I didn't know yet was that before the 1960s, most people with a heroin habit *did* get it from the pharmacy. But Thatcher's austerity, the global drug war and doctors' preference for methadone had squeezed the program down to only a few hundred patients. They got their heroin prescribed at clinics in Manchester and Liverpool or at a hospital in South London. Nobody new was getting in.

Our conversation ended abruptly when a guy with a shaved head and tweed sports jacket slid in the door. Skinny was here at last.

I had been in London about three weeks when classes started. Even if I was still using, I was going to school. That part of my plan hadn't changed. But the LSE was not what I thought. I pictured an austere, academic environment with soaring oak trees, old stone buildings and wood panelling, but you could easily miss the compact urban campus. It was down a tiny lane, right off the Strand in Central London. A warren of little concrete passages connected a dozen mid-century buildings, all crammed around a central alleyway. The Three Tuns student pub sold subsidized pints for one pound each. There were only about twelve other students in my program. We took seminars on the theories of power, the rise of nationalism and global patterns of wealth distribution. It was heady stuff, but I managed to follow it. The profs just talked. They rarely used the blackboard or other visuals.

I was given a small office in the British Library of Political and Economic Science—one of the largest social sciences libraries in the world. Karl Marx had studied there, and staff claimed that his ghost still haunted the basement stacks, but I never saw him.

Using a library was difficult. I couldn't see the computer screens or the little call numbers on the spines of books. But friends and staff helped me find what I was looking for. I slowly assembled the information I needed to write my master's thesis. My tiny office had a leaded window and a clanking radiator. But it was cozy and all mine. The library was open late, and I worked on my thesis at night, taking the occasional break to fix. I tried to put my words into an academic voice, not the style of a socialist newspaper or punk lyrics. I was writing about the globalization of capitalism and the demise of the welfare state. As transnational corporations got stronger, governments were hurrying to get out of their way, cutting social programs and deregulating economies. We were on the way to a very bleak future, I wrote.

I moved out of Central London and into a flat with two roommates in Stamford Hill in Hackney, coming back to my office to write. Heroin suppressed my appetite, so for months I ate little else than small cups of chocolate pudding. I grew thin and gaunt. Sunny and I would pool our cash to buy in bulk off Skinny. One night it was Sunny's turn to make the run, but he never came back. I called him a hundred times, worried that he'd overdosed or been arrested. A few weeks later, he called to apologize. He'd done all our dope then checked himself into rehab. He promised to pay me back someday.

My friend Molly lived nearby. She was a recreational heroin user—a chipper, a dabbler. Molly could take it or leave it. She'd do heroin as a kind of special treat. There were plenty of people like Molly who enjoyed heroin but just never got wired. I wished I could take it or leave it. But I couldn't leave it.

One Friday night Molly stopped by. She was already a few pints in when she plonked down on my mattress and started to make up a hit. EDM blasted from my upstairs neighbour. He was a DJ, and the throbbing ceiling was part of every weekend. I looked out onto the darkness of Thorpe Road. At the end of our street, the last train of the night thundered past. I looked back into the room, and she wasn't moving. I shook her. She was out cold, rig still in her hand.

I searched for a pulse, but all I felt was my own heart, pounding like a piledriver. I yelled at her, pinched her. Her lips were turning blue. My head tingled as I started CPR—I felt like I wasn't getting any oxygen either. I had brought back overdoses from the edge before, but I could tell this one was worse. She was far gone, falling over the edge.

We had no phone, so I carried her out of the flat over my shoulder, like a firefighter. I hauled Molly down the street as a nauseating vertigo built inside me. A group of creepy lager lads cheered at the sight of a guy carrying what looked like a passed-out drunk girl. I leaned her against a call box and stabbed out the UK number for emergency services: 999.

My future flashed ahead. Molly dead, me arrested and sent off to some ancient British prison. HMP Wormwood Scrubs. Strangeways, here we come. Across the planet, but doing the same shit I'd done eight time zones to the west.

"What service, please?" a woman answered, all treble and buzzing phone line. She could have been calling announcements on the Tube. Her aggressively calm tone mocked my panic.

"I think my friend is overdosing!" I blurted, my voice dancing up the minor scale with each syllable. Molly was a lightweight but could never admit it.

"Chill out, man," came a deeper, groggy, slurred response.

"Overdose! I think my friend is overdosing!" I shouted, confused and repeating myself.

But the slurring didn't come from the earpiece. It came from Molly, eyes still shut.

"Jesus fucking Christ!" I shouted down the line, at the sky and at Molly, and hung up the phone. I slumped down on the pavement and let her crumple down with me. The Friday night revellers paid us little mind.

"Relax, Garth," Molly slurred. Relief flooded over me.

Molly had no memory of the last ten minutes. She didn't understand what I was so upset about, and she seemed determined to learn nothing from the night's events.

With Molly's arm around my neck, we stumbled back to my room. I put her on the bed. I knew I was going to have to keep a close eye on her for the rest of the night. The stress of the near miss had burned through every opioid molecule in my bloodstream, so I started preparing a hit for myself. It never occurred to me that I was taking the same risk. "Make me one too," she mumbled from the bed.

I shook my head. Fuck that. And I swore to myself that I'd never do dope with a weekend warrior ever again.

Hundred Block Rock

t was a crisp November day in Vancouver. I looked out the bus window as the grey of East Van slowly gave way to the colourful autumn leaves of the University of British Columbia. There was a good chance I could be arrested today, so I made sure I had nothing illegal in my pockets.

I had moved back from London several months before, broke and in the middle of a historic snowstorm. I had a master's degree, but I needed money right away, so I shovelled snow for cash and worked for my uncle Buck's construction outfit for a few weeks. I got on welfare and looked for jobs. I still wanted to leave heroin behind, but I realized that I could keep my habit under wraps and continue working in social movements.

When I got off the bus at the campus, police and security people were swarming everywhere. They were protecting the eighteen world leaders and various other dignitaries who'd flown in for the 1997 Asia-Pacific Economic Cooperation summit. A sea of activists representing groups from around the city was assembling by the Student Union Building. I was one of the organizers with a socialist group from East Van. We opposed APEC because it was part of a series of trade negotiations that were handing over more power to transnational corporations at the expense of workers, Indigenous people, the environment and human rights. It was the kind of theft on a global scale that I'd studied at LSE.

Protesters milled around, chatting. I wrote the number of a lawyer on my arm in marker—to call in case of arrest. We expected trouble. One of the other leaders, Jaggi Singh, had already been arrested the day before. He was snatched by cops while walking across campus. A group called APEC Alert had spent weeks preparing—holding meetings, making signs and strategizing actions. Some activists had been camped out in tents for several days. Police had been spying on us the whole time. The RCMP distributed info sheets among their frontline officers, identifying "ringleaders"—including me.

About 1,500 of us marched toward where the summit was being held, in the Museum of Anthropology. We made our way down a long, open boulevard, chanting slogans, waving banners and banging drums. The RCMP were ready to meet us—a solid line of dark uniforms and another line of bicycle cops in hi-vis jackets. They stood in columns, protected by a chain-link fence. Tension crackled in the air between the two sides.

As we reached the cops, I felt a surge of adrenaline—I had no idea what was going to happen. This was it. I took my place with other organizers, near the front. My heart was pounding, but I tried to project confidence to those behind me. Through a megaphone, I warned protesters if we got any closer, we'd all risk arrest. A cheer went up. Everyone knew the stakes. We chanted louder. Through binoculars, I could see snipers in position on the roof of the Chan Centre auditorium. *Are they willing to shoot us?*

Then things escalated fast. I could see the front of the march arriving at the fence. A few students climbed up on the concrete footing and grabbed on to the chain link for support. The fence buckled. A cheer went up. There was no plan to march past this point. We were still half a kilometre from where world leaders were meeting.

I heard the hiss as a cop fired a fat stream of pepper spray into the march. The acrid smell filled the air. Protesters fell back, some moving aimlessly as if blinded, some struggling for breath. Cops stormed into us, grabbing protesters and rushing them back behind the police lines. Some cops wrestled protesters to the ground and dragged them off. I picked up a guy who'd got knocked down.

People chanted "Shame! Shame Shame!" and police dogs barked. I had been in situations like this before. I stood my ground and remained calm. I poured water on my bandana and tied it over my mouth and nose.

A line of Mounties advanced into us. Blasts of pepper spray swept across the crowd. My throat and eyes burned. I stumbled back, streaming tears and coughing. Luckily, the bandana had blocked much of the pepper spray. I had to stay focused so I could help others to retreat in an orderly fashion. Amidst all the coughing and yelling, I heard a familiar voice. A woman named Andy hollered as she was being dragged away by two cops. Andy was one of the bravest among us, always on the front lines. I shouted her name, but my voice was lost in the tumult.

When I finally got home that night, I was exhausted, my eyes still stinging and my clothes covered in pepper spray. I was angry but also proud. I felt confident in my role as an organizer that day. I called the lawyers' office. People were slowly getting released, although all the women had been needlessly strip-searched. On TV, Prime Minister Jean Chrétien was asked about cops using pepper spray on protesters. He seemed confused and quipped, "For me, pepper, I put it on my plate."

About six months later, Andy and I started dating. Andy had a sharp intellect, massive vocabulary and was full of energy. We were both part of a new organization that was trying to take the police to task for their spying, assaults and arrests at APEC. On our first date, I told Andy about my dope habit and she didn't judge me.

There were always meetings, talks, postering, demonstrations, phone calls and articles to write. A few of us from that protest were interviewed by the media. We became minor public figures in Canada. People recognized me on the street. I worried some enterprising reporter would figure out I was wired and expose me. And I worried that I'd be judged and mistrusted by the movement if they knew about my habit. It wasn't always explicit. It was mostly just a vibe, although one squat in East Vancouver established a "no junkies" rule. So I kept quiet.

Then Andy saw a poster for a rally about overdoses. She said we should go. "I'd rather do dope than hold up signs about it," I joked, trying to change the subject. I didn't want to think of myself as an addict. I still planned to kick, so there was no point getting involved. To me, heroin was a medication, not an entire identity. I didn't want all the TV and movie stereotypes attached to me. I didn't want to be thought of as dirty, untrustworthy and violent. But Andy was stubborn, so we headed out to the rally. Even with all the pepper spray, I had been a lot more comfortable at the APEC protests.

The familiar old buildings, pawn shops and greasy spoons of the Downtown Eastside were a welcome reprieve from the glass condo towers and hipster cafés that had been eating away at the rest of Vancouver while I was in London. I knew these cracked and rutted streets like old veins. Hastings, Columbia, Carrall, Main, Dunlevy. The wall of blue-grey North Shore Mountains appeared to lift straight up behind the rundown old hotels. Burrard Inlet lay between, changing colour like a mood ring: blue, green, grey, black. Just a couple of blocks away, the port's red gantry cranes stooped over container ships, hungry mechanical giraffes, feeding all night. The ghosts of generations of resource workers still haunted the neighbourhood's small rooms.

Everyone was meeting up near Main and Hastings. A small group was congregating on the corner with some signs, banners and a megaphone. A black plywood coffin stood on its end. Hand-printed signs read, "Drug users are people too," "Who's the next overdose victim?" and "Stop police harassment." An ambulance roared past us, sirens blaring. There were a lot more sirens since I got back.

Fatal overdoses from China White were surging in BC, and the crisis had exploded out of East Vancouver and into the mainstream. Politicians and journalists were talking about "the drug problem," cops were everywhere, and the Vancouver/Richmond Health Board had declared a public health emergency. It was estimated that four hundred might die in 1998, a significant increase. The trend line was heading in an ominous direction. Drug users just weren't used to this high-potency dope. We often didn't have the tolerance.

HIV was spreading faster here than anywhere outside sub-Saharan Africa, and it was spreading through our rigs. New syringes were still scarce, and making matters worse, shooting coke was taking off. Since the rush of cocaine is short-lived, people were injecting more frequently and going through more needles.

There were no supervised injection sites. Naloxone—the overdose-reversing medication—could only be accessed by medical professionals. Methadone maintenance treatment was limited. And every week, I heard about somebody else who had died, including my friend Nick. Some part of me knew I could be next.

There was a nervous energy at the march. Some people seemed ready to slip down an alley and blow the whole thing off. In such an over-policed neighbourhood, why do something that will attract more heat? We stood on the sidewalk, shifting around, afraid to take the street.

Then Andy started a chant. I was trying to keep a low profile—which isn't easy for a six-foot-four albino with a hollering girlfriend.

"We're here! We're high! Get used to it!" Andy yelled, pumping her fist with each phrase, her voice ringing down the block. She was borrowing an old ACT UP/Queer Nation chant popularized by HIV/AIDS activists, "We're here. We're queer. Get used to it!" Andy had marched in plenty of those actions.

Another loud voice joined Andy's. Ann Livingston took up the chant, with a laugh in her voice. Ann was an activist I recognized from meetings and workshops at La Quena, a café on Commercial Drive where the original plans for a drug user union first started brewing. East Van was bubbling with leftist groups, socialist study circles and communist sects from around the globe. In halls, homes and coffee shops, people were planning to change the world. Everything was up for debate. Ann herself was not a drug user, but she lived on the Downtown Eastside, had noticed all the sirens recently and started getting involved.

Andy's and Ann's chant had broken the tension, and people laughed. One by one, then en masse, we took the street. It felt amazing—a legion of drug users—not embarrassed or ashamed, but proudly marching and chanting slogans.

The Downtown Eastside was like a small town. Everybody knew each other. We marched down Hastings, past Columbia and Carrall, then back past Main, Gore and Dunlevy. We marched past grandly named hotels that were now cheap rooming houses: the Balmoral, the Roosevelt, the Regent. It was hard to imagine this place back in the early twentieth century, when it was the pulsing neon downtown core of the city, full of shops, theatres and restaurants.

We stopped marching and the chanting died down. A speaker took the mic to call out the mayor for a lack of action on the overdose deaths, called for detox on demand and said we needed prescription heroin, just like they used to have in the UK. I found myself cheering along with everyone else.

Community leader Bud Osborn was then introduced. I'd been at other demonstrations where Bud read his poetry, but I hadn't ever heard him talk. Bud was originally from Ohio and came to Canada to avoid the draft. He had been to university, was a published poet and had a dope habit. With his glasses and longish curly brown hair, collared shirt and baggy sweater, he was exactly my idea of a poet.

Bud took the mic. He talked about the deaths. He said we needed a safe injection site. That's why he'd talked his way into getting appointed to the Vancouver/Richmond Health Board, he explained. I was very impressed. I had never heard of an official body like the Health Board listening to an intravenous drug user, never mind inviting one of us to join. The only way I have ever gotten into rooms like that was by disguising the fact that I used drugs. Bud practically put it on his resumé.

This demonstration was part of a campaign, Bud explained. Last year, activists pulled a chain across Hastings and blocked traffic. They had a banner that read, "THE KILLING FIELDS." At Oppenheimer Park, Bud and other activists had planted one thousand white crosses to represent everyone who had died of overdose in the previous five years. Bud's poem "Hundred Block Rock" spoke to the grim mood of the moment.

hundred block rock
shoot up shock
police chief
cold grief
war on drugs

pull the plug
clean it up
nowhere to go
ground zero
overload jail
rock and wail
where a dopefiend stood
coming soon
to your neighbourhood

I had been in Bud's position before, at other demonstrations for other causes. I had been an organizer, standing at the front with a mic and intelligent words to share. But I didn't have Bud's bravery. I shied away from saying "I'm an addict" at an Anonymous twelve-step meeting; I couldn't imagine saying it through a microphone, in front of the media. But Bud didn't care if the world dismissed him as a junkie. Hell, he was even redefining people's idea of what a junkie was. Bud gave us a new way to describe ourselves. Through his poetry, Bud reclaimed the old media slur "dopefiend." He liberated it from those hackneyed moral panic articles and handed it back to us. "Dopefiend" had a kind of old-timey charm to it. It felt much better than "junkie," "addict" or "crackhead."

When I wasn't with other drug users or close friends, I tried to keep my habit a secret. I often used alone. I wore long sleeves in summer, pulling them over my wrists as the track marks crept down my arms and onto my hands. Yet the people organizing this demonstration weren't hiding. They were fighting for their rights—and mine too—unashamed and knowing full well they could be targeted by the cops or the press. It was inspiring, but I wasn't brave like them. And I hated that.

Politicians' solutions to the "drug problem" always focused on what *we* should do. Quit. Get clean. Work the steps. Accept responsibility. Pull yourself up by your bootstraps. It all sounded simple to an outsider, but it isn't so easy. Reading off a piece of paper, another speaker said, "For a lot of us, kicking dope might take years." I nodded. It was taking me years. He continued, "And for some, it might never happen. That shouldn't be a death sentence."

His statement was like a bolt of lightning to my skull. It was so obvious. Some people just couldn't kick. Part of me worried that I might be one of them. Maybe it was just as important to keep people alive as it was to get them clean.

Having no sanctioned supervised injection sites meant the city was one massive unsupervised injection site. I used in an empty apartment in my dealer's building, or in an alley, or in a McDonald's bathroom, or in a boarded-up abandoned building popped open to use as a shooting gallery.

Some people wanted to change things. As a teenage drug user, I received my first new syringes thanks to the efforts of activists like John Turvey, a former drug user who handed out syringes illegally from a backpack. Turvey started the Downtown Eastside Youth Activities Society, which opened a storefront needle exchange.

On my first visit there, I had to roll up my sleeve and show my track marks to prove I was a drug user. I was registered as GRM and would tell them my handle each time I came back.

I had to give over my old spike to receive a new one. This strict exchange system was set up as a defensive response against the many critics who said needles shouldn't be given out at all. This meant I wasn't allowed to take a dozen for later or for friends. Plenty of drug users didn't want to be seen at a place like this, and so they couldn't access the clean needles. As a result, the number of rigs in circulation was kept low.

Some activists argued that we couldn't wait for the government, we'd have to do it ourselves. Ann Livingston told me about the "Back Alley," an unsanctioned safe injection site that was running for a short time while I was in London. Ann, William Kay, Melissa Eror and a few drug users opened the site in a rented storefront at 356 Powell Street, near Oppenheimer Park. They did not ask for permission.

Meetings were held in the front room, where there was a desk, a table, couches and coffee. In the back room there were three booths for injecting. To keep the peace with the cops, the group made a rule that there could be no dealing in the space. People soon covered the walls with murals and poetry, like this:

Sleep with the sun
Rise with the moon
I feel all right
With my needle & spoon

The no-dealing rule was hard to enforce. There were always a couple of assholes who didn't care if their short-term greed ruined a good thing for everyone else. Within a few months, police raided the Back Alley and it was forced to close. But Ann,

Melissa and others were already thinking about another project. They held meetings in Oppenheimer Park where drug users talked about forming a union. It would ultimately be called the Vancouver Area Network of Drug Users.

Andy and I said goodbye to Ann and Bud and walked down the street. Andy caught a bus and I kept walking, without a destination in mind. I thought about John Turvey's needle backpack and Ann Livingston and the unsanctioned supervised injection site. Doing these things saved lives but was totally illegal. These were the same kind of law-breaking civil disobedience tactics we used in other movements to resist the march of global capitalism at trade summits around the world. They were the same tactics that movements had been using for centuries. Disobeying unjust laws. I was starting to understand the drug war in a different light.

It was hard to quit. The last decade of my life was proof of that. Instead of insisting on abstinence like twelve-step meetings, the demonstration called for programs that could reduce the harms of drug use. Programs that could save lives. It made so much sense. I wanted to join up and march under that banner. But I just couldn't accept that that was who I was. I couldn't admit that I was a dopefiend.

Gonna Kick Tomorrow

My fingers ached to dial the number. They knew it by muscle memory. Like a scale, spidering up and down the keypad. A ten-note musical phrase I hummed to myself on a loop. Dope was always just one call away. Beep beep beep.

The newspapers called it "dial-a-dope." But I just called him Lee. Unlike Skinny, Lee had no habit to support. He never touched drugs. It was strictly a business thing. I'd call Lee up and say the code—"One Q"—and one of Lee's drivers would arrive at my place faster than a pizza delivery. The heroin was always the same: it was strong and cooked up clean. It had legs enough to keep me well for twelve hours or more. Lee always weighed his shit out properly, never trying to short me. He was open from nine a.m. to nine p.m.—every single day. Including New Year's and Christmas.

Sometimes Lee would deliver the dope himself. He'd roll up in an Audi or some other rented luxury car, its interior always spotless. He wore polo shirts, always with a phone clipped to his belt, and glasses with a transitioning tint that always seemed a few steps behind local light conditions. He was kind too. Once he brought some toys for my cat. Another time, after a major bust threw the city into a heroin drought, Lee warned Jeff and me that the price for down had doubled and the quality was low. "Don't buy this," he advised us frankly. We had no choice and bought some anyway. But Lee was right. It was garbage.

Buying heroin from Lee was smooth. Effortless. And with each call, my habit grew. My first smash, back in San Francisco, was less than half a point—about a twentieth of a gram—and it had filled me with a warm, euphoric sense of belonging. Now I was injecting nearly a gram a day—costing over a hundred dollars—and it wasn't even getting me high anymore. It just treated the dopesickness.

I owed my friends, acquaintances and dealers money. And almost every dollar I made was going up my arm. I got freelance writing gigs, sometimes for the *Vancouver Sun*. Grand Chief Doug Kelly hired me to research and write a major paper arguing for First Nation control over health care systems. I worked as a day labourer in construction. I was an extra for movies and TV shows made in Vancouver, like *Rumble in the Bronx*, *The X-Files* and *Da Vinci's Inquest*. But I could only hold down short-term gigs. When we were dopesick and desperate, Jeff and I had a scheme rehabilitating used computer equipment. I had another involving cartons of cigarettes. I knew we might get busted, but I didn't know what else to do. I'm not sure when I realized the honeymoon was over—it didn't happen all at once. But eventually it was unmistakable: heroin was ruining every part of my life.

At night, I walked around East Vancouver. Down to the port, across the tracks, along Hastings Street, up to Trout Lake. Bats, coyotes, raccoons, car thieves, sex workers and graveyard-shift clerks ignored me and went about their business. Sometimes Jeff and I sat by the water in CRAB Park, talking for hours or just watching the freighters on Burrard Inlet.

The everyday cycle of dopesickness, grinding for cash and using took all of my energy. I found it nearly impossible to meet any other kind of commitment outside of work. I couldn't make regular rehearsals, so I wasn't in a band. I turned down invitations from friends to go to parties or the movies. I was a no-show for family events. My sister started calling me "the king of bail." I isolated myself from most people who didn't use heroin.

No dope meant no sleep. I'd lie awake watching headlights from passing cars illuminate my shredded curtains. My apartment was pitch black because I hadn't paid the electricity bill. I hadn't paid my phone bill either. An eviction notice was taped to my door. When was the last time I made food? Or ate? I could smell the drain in the kitchen. Dirty dishes in the sink. Used needles lay in ranks on the table, waiting to be dropped off at the needle depot. Black mould was creeping up the wall, like the self-pity that smothered my life.

When I did sleep, I dreamed of dying. When I was awake, I longed for oblivion. Not death, just nothingness.

Even my body seemed to be in total revolt. I'd worked my way up and down the veins of both arms. Pipelines that once lay on the surface retreated underground, hiding from the spike. I was covered in scars. I had an abscess on my left hand and golf balls under my skin from where I'd missed while injecting. I wore my work clothes from construction gigs. They were threadbare and unfashionable. I couldn't afford style. I felt old and exhausted. I was too thin. A couple dozen friends had already died of overdose. I felt like I wouldn't survive this.

Heroin had been my saviour. It used to provide relief. It had made me feel good about myself, but it wasn't working anymore. I was just left with all the risks—overdose, arrest, dopesickness and poverty. I felt betrayed but I knew I only had myself to blame. I was desperate to quit. But how? I couldn't face kicking cold turkey again, like in London, shitting and shaking, the darkness coming over me. In a flash, I remembered standing in the bathroom. I could feel that knife in my hand with its serrated edge and wanting to punch a hole in my skin to let the sick out. I shook my head. I'd tried to kick over a dozen times since London. Sometimes I had a plan. Sometimes I was just out of money and dope. But I never made it more than a couple of days. I knew I wouldn't be able to do it alone.

A powerful fantasy bloomed in my desperation. I imagined some kind of recovery facility—like a BC version of the Betty Ford Center. I'd walk in the door and submit myself completely to whatever program they were peddling. It would be a clean place with clean sheets and clean food. There'd be music therapy. I could try to get better at guitar. Maybe they'd even have equine therapy. I'd heard about that. I liked horses, though to be honest, I had no clue how horses were supposed to help you quit dope. There'd be mountains and meadows and cabins. And expert doctors with all the answers. I'd be born again clean.

If I was going to make this dream a reality, there was a step I had to take. It was something I'd resisted all this time—even in my most desperate moments. I'd managed to create a protective bubble around my family. I cleaned myself up when I went to visit. I shielded them from the worst parts of my life. They didn't know about Victoria or that I'd done sex work. I lied, telling them I was clean when I wasn't. But I never stole from them. When the whole family pitched in to help me pay for my LSE tuition, I didn't spend it on dope. But now I knew I needed their help. And so I called my mother. I decided to talk quickly, so I couldn't back out.

"Mom, I have this plan to get help. There's a place, I think, and it's not too expensive. I know this one guy who went and he's doing better." I was babbling. I imagined cutting the copper phone lines to stop the signal. "And if it works out, I can get healthy and make some positive changes . . ." I trailed off.

"Where is this rehab?" Mom asked, suspiciously.

I thought about those mountains and said, "Umm, somewhere near Squamish, I think. I'll have to check." I was vague about the details. I turned my lighter over in my pocket, feeling its smooth sides. I was in my late twenties and asking my mother for money. It was humiliating, but the deceit was the worst part. I felt like I was selling her a used car.

She was quiet for a moment. "How do I know I wouldn't be funding a drug habit instead of recovery?"

She was right. Her money would probably go right up my arm before I got anywhere near a recovery house. The lie was like an eel in my stomach. If I had a legitimate plan, I'm pretty sure she would have helped me. But I wanted to shield my mother from my seedy, ugly life as much as I wanted to tell her everything. I wanted to tell her how bad my habit was—much worse than I had let on. I wanted to tell her the things I'd done to pay for dope. I winced at the memory of shooting dope in her bathroom and leaving specks of blood in the sink. I wanted to apologize and tell her that the world she lived in didn't want me. I didn't know how to fit myself into it. I had tried. I wanted to apologize for not being the son she hoped for. But I couldn't explain. And so, like many times before, I said nothing while the line hummed in our long silence. I felt like we'd been sharing these silences since I was a kid. I said goodbye and hung up without asking further about money.

Fuck rehab anyway. And all the judgy recovery zealots. "Oh hey, Garth! Thirty-three days clean!" I remembered the bearded guy everybody called Jay, fresh from rehab, rosy-faced and several pounds heavier. I'd never begrudge Jay his pink cloud. But I didn't need his prideful smiles and slogans at the ready, right out of the Big Book. He was back in the hood, looking to complete that last step—Step 12: "carry the message to the addict who still suffers."

I'd known plenty of people like Jay, floating in like Christian missionaries to save us sinners. Fresh from some recovery program, colourful clean-time key fobs dangling from their belt loops. Back on the block to share the good news—and maybe one last shameful hit. But after months of rehab, their tolerance was shot, and it often really was their last hit.

I was considering desperate options now. And one of those options was methadone. Methadone is a synthetic opioid. It does not come from the opium poppy. I'd taken it a couple of times in a pinch. It kept dopesickness at bay and lasted much longer than heroin—often keeping me well for an entire day. But everyone said methadone is harder to kick than heroin.

The formulation of methadone we have in North America is an agonist that fights euphoria. Even though methadone is an opioid, it doesn't really give you that "warm hug" feeling like heroin—unless you take a bunch. Worse, methadone blocks the euphoric effects of other opioids you might use in addition to it. If you're on methadone, you have to use even more heroin to feel anything at all. That's the main thing methadone tries to do. No highs, no lows. Just an even, straight line of bland wellness.

One of the world's first methadone clinics opened in Vancouver, in 1959. Like most innovations in drug policy, it began as a small pilot project. Dr. Robert Halliday first tried to open his clinic in Kitsilano, but local residents responded with what one newspaper called "a storm of protest." Residents claimed property values would fall and the streets wouldn't be safe. Eventually, a site was found near the Vancouver General Hospital. Dr. Halliday planned to use methadone to quickly taper his patients down to abstinence over twelve days. But he soon figured out this wasn't as effective as allowing patients to stay on ongoing maintenance doses.

In a 1967 study, Dr. Halliday sought to measure "improvement in a specific area" rather than "abstention from drugs" only. He found that 43 per cent of his study subjects showed some overall improvement in "drug use, work, criminal behaviour, community associations, friendship patterns and family relationships." That's still less than half, and they didn't get off drugs. But Halliday could see that access to an affordable supply of regulated opioids could make all the difference.

Like a lot of drug users, I had a pretty low opinion of the methadone program. It seemed like the end of the line. Methadone was for people who couldn't get themselves clean or hack the daily grind of life as a dopefiend. Musicians like Billie Holiday, Charlie Parker, Sid Vicious, Kurt Cobain and Lou Reed used heroin. But there was nothing cool about methadone. Nobody said methadone was the creative engine behind their amazing records. You weren't partying when you took it. You were sitting around a sad waiting room full of other patients. And there was no exit plan for getting clean. No freedom date. You were parked on the program, where you could languish forever. I guess that's why people called it liquid handcuffs.

"Methadone is only for real fuck-ups," an old-timer once told me. "You gotta have a bad habit. Real bad. For years and years, like me, or they won't let you on it. You, you're too young," he said, pointing at me. "But you're getting there."

I'm not going to stay *on methadone,* I reassured myself. *I'm just gonna use it to get clean.* My plan was to get on the program so that I'd have a relatively affordable supply of opioids to keep me from getting dopesick. Then I'd ask them to taper me down to nothing. It felt like a smarter plan than trying to go cold turkey by myself again. This time I'd have medication to help.

I asked around and was recommended a clinic on Hastings and Princess. I made sure I wasn't dopesick on the day I went in. When I met the doctor, I told him how serious I was about recovery. How hard I was willing to work. How capable I was. But my plan backfired. Instead of telling him how much effort I was going to put in, I should have told him how desperate I was. After a quick conversation, the doctor said he had decided to reject my request. "If I let you on the program," he said, "I'll have to turn away someone who needs it more, like a sex worker." I hadn't mentioned my previous sex work. He never asked. I wasn't sure what I was supposed to say. I didn't realize that spaces on the program were so strictly rationed, even as bodies piled up from overdoses and HIV, and I truly didn't want to take away a place from someone who needed it more. Maybe I didn't deserve to be on their program. *Fuck this,* I said to myself as I walked home empty-handed. *I'll have to do it myself. I'll have to go see Simon.*

I was now living at the Georgia Estates, a grand name for a disintegrating stucco three-storey walk-up apartment building where a feral band of twelve-year-olds roamed the property looking to rob visitors. Across the hall from my apartment lived Simon, a small-time heroin dealer who sold to support his own habit. Simon also sold methadone that he bought off patients who were on the program. I figured he'd be able to sell me some.

"Mornin', Garth." Simon answered the door in Adidas tear-away track pants and a white tank top with little burn holes down the front. Simon was imposingly tall and lanky, and always dressed in athletic gear, though I never saw him play any sports. Then again, I wore a motorcycle jacket but had no Harley. Simon's wife, a no-nonsense small-town Alberta woman, said hello to me from somewhere inside.

"Got methadone?" I asked.

"Oh yeah, sure," Simon said, turning toward his fridge. "I sell the cure as well as the disease." I chuckled politely as Simon pulled out a translucent plastic bottle with the prescription label scratched off.

"How much do ya want?" he asked.

I knew exactly the quantity I needed. "One hundred milli-litres," I answered.

I gave Simon my last twenty-five bucks and he gave me the bottle. I went back across the hall and checked my supplies for the coming days: radio, two packages of Camel cigarettes, Kurt Vonnegut novel, container of Aunt Rose's chicken corn soup, box of Cap'n Crunch cereal and six cups of Kozy Shack rice pudding. I didn't want to leave the apartment for any reason. Finally, I consulted the hopeful little plan I had written down in my notebook:

> Day 1—40ml
> Day 2—30ml
> Day 3—20ml
> Day 4—10ml
> Day 5—0ml—Clean!

I looked at the word "clean" on the bottom of the page. Getting clean had been my goal for ages, always just over the horizon. But the word had a kind of backhanded slap to it. All those twelve-step terms seemed to. If I wasn't clean, I must be dirty. "Find a new word," I wrote in my notebook, before snapping it shut. I measured out the first dose of forty millilitres, knocked it back and waited.

I chain-smoked and watched reruns of daytime TV for about an hour, then I took another twenty millilitres and tried to go to sleep. The next day I got up and finished the bottle. My plan was out the window. All the methadone was gone, and I was getting restless and twitchy. I paced my room. This wasn't going to work. I walked back across the hall and asked Simon to front me a quarter of his "disease." He wasn't surprised to see me but had the good manners not to mention it.

My family gathered at the Women's Hospital. I was in long sleeves to hide my track marks. My sister was about to give birth. She laughed in the dimly lit delivery room and said, "Just get it out of me!" She'd brought a boom box and was playing Pink Floyd. When we were kids, we cranked *The Dark Side of the Moon* in our parents' basement. Gill had always wanted to be a mother. I was excited for her.

Outside, my brother-in-law, Chas, paced in the ambulance bay, all jitters and nerves. "I don't like hospitals," he muttered to me. I knew why. Chas was Cree, from the Peguis First Nation in Manitoba. Social workers had seized babies from Peguis families—as they had from Indigenous families across Canada, for decades. Jeff was seized when he was only a few months old. Sometimes the babies were taken right at the hospital. Dad clapped a hand on Chas's shoulder to reassure him.

A couple of hours later, Paige was born. Dad and I went into Gill's room. She was exhausted but happy, cuddling the tiny newborn against her. Gill asked me if I wanted to hold her. Paige was swaddled in a little white blanket, her head in a hospital baby cap. It was easy to see her in the dimly lit room. Paige was calm and trusting in my arms. She looked up at me and our eyes locked. I felt an immediate, intense connection, like someone just plugged in a patch cord between us. It wasn't like anything I'd felt before. The feeling sliced clean through the seedy clutter and shame of my life. I loved her. I needed to be ready to do my part to help raise her. I told her quietly that I wanted a better world for her. I wanted to get better too.

But those good feelings curdled on my way back home. When I got there, I started gouging away with a needle, searching, probing for a vein. My radio was on in the background. A news anchor mocked my frustrated efforts to find a vein: "Wall Street is feeling ebullient under President Bush . . ."

Sludgy blood crawled down my arm, over my shirt, my jeans, the table and floor. Finding a vein had been taking longer and longer these past months, and now I had used up all the tiny veins on my hands and feet. I'd even used my jugular once. My veins were blown out. My body was refusing to let in the heroin it needed.

Sitting there, staring at the bright red blood flecks, I felt a wave of guilt. I was breaking a commitment I'd just made to a ten-minute-old baby. I put my head down on the table and cried out frustrated, exhausted tears.

When I came to, I pulled the plunger out and tipped the column of bloody sludge down my throat. The dirty metallic taste of blood reminded me of all the times I'd been punched in the mouth. I slipped under the covers with Andy, who had long since gone to bed. The wool army blanket was scratchy and full of burn holes from when she'd fallen asleep while smoking. Even a screaming smoke alarm was not enough to rouse her. It was the new millennium, but it felt like I'd been left behind in the old one. I was thirty. I felt ancient and out of touch.

The sun would be up in an hour or so. The guy on the radio lost his confident news presenter voice, shakily explaining that planes had struck both World Trade Center towers. Within weeks, our global anti-capitalist movement and its dreams of a new world would be cancelled. World leaders were leaving trade negotiations to the bureaucrats and preparing for war. Legislatures and parliaments were drawing up rights-limiting anti-terrorism laws. Boots were kicking in doors all over the planet. The world's future was being recalibrated. I had to recalibrate my future too. Andy and I were heading in different directions. We'd hang on for a while longer, but ultimately, the relationship was doomed. Change was in the air. I had to make good my promise to my newborn niece. I called my sister. Hearing the new baby gurgling in the background, I asked, "How's Paige?"

I sat at the back of the number 9 bus, watching rain bead across the window. Simon had written down an address for me: 750 West Broadway. It was a methadone clinic.

Its generic name, "Bio-Scan," seemed designed to give nothing away about the kind of medical service provided there. The clinic was on the tenth floor of a bland, 1960s-era office building in a long city block of obscure medical specialists. Inside, it felt like a cross between a doctor's waiting room and a probation office.

I approached the receptionist. She asked me to fill out some paperwork, then handed me a specimen cup with my name printed on the lid. "Please return this afterward," she said, and instructed me to leave my jacket and bag behind as

I headed to the bathroom. That was a clinic rule designed to prevent us from trying to fool urinalysis by smuggling in someone else's piss.

After filling the cup, I turned on the hot water tap to wash my hands, but only cold water came out. I'd later learn that this was another measure put in place to keep us from trying to pass someone else's piss off as our own: they didn't want us to warm up cold urine in the sink. I put my filled specimen cup on the receptionist's desk. She put on gloves and checked it with a thermometer. She told me that they were going to send the cup to a lab to make sure I tested positive for heroin. They wanted to be sure I was fucked up enough to be on the program.

A middle-aged woman with glasses, short curly brown hair and an Austrian accent called my name, and I followed her into a little examination room. Dr. M took my medical history and had me stand on a scale. I was very thin—all ribs and elbows. "Like sleeping with a bag of antlers," a girlfriend once told me. My fashion wasn't helping. I had pawned my leather jacket and only had somebody else's comically large maroon coat left to wear, accentuating my emaciated frame. I knew I looked bad and I wondered what Dr. M thought of me. When she finished examining me, she said she was going to order blood tests for hepatitis C and HIV. Suddenly I realized I hadn't been tested for several years. I felt a wave of anxiety about what those tests might reveal.

With the formalities out of the way, Dr. M gave me her philosophy on addiction, which she said was based on overwhelming medical consensus. She told me that addiction is a "chronic, relapsing disorder." "Disorder" meant that it was serious, and life-threatening. But it also meant that Dr. M didn't see my addiction as being my fault. I was just wired wrong. "Chronic" meant that no matter how hard I worked, I was always going to be an "addict." My addiction would be with me forever, and the best I could hope to do was treat it. "Relapsing" meant that these treatments were likely to fail from time to time. Eventually I'd fall off the horse.

Some of what Dr. M was saying resonated with me. I definitely preferred to think of addiction as a disease rather than a moral failing. But I already had one lifelong genetic disorder— albinism. And it was depressing to think I was stuck with another. I wondered if I could really do anything to change my fate, or if I'd just be a congenital fuck-up for life. I didn't want to be on methadone for years and years, but I knew I'd need to be on it for more than four days, like I'd tried with Simon's juice. My new plan was to get on the program, but only for a few months. Once I was totally clear of opioids, I could start a band, or go back to school or get a full-time job. I could pursue a future.

Since I still was a novice about methadone, I didn't really understand how this other drug was supposed to "treat" my heroin addiction. Later, Dr. M would explain it to me.

She took out a piece of paper and began drawing a graph. Across the bottom she sketched a horizontal line, representing the twenty-four hours in a day. Then she drew a vertical line up the left margin of the page, representing the level of drugs in your system. She wrote "withdrawal" at the bottom of the vertical line and "high" at the top. Then Dr. M drew a red line across the graph, dramatically swooping up and down—from the despair of dopesickness to the warm euphoric hug of dope, and back to withdrawal again. At the end of the graph, she shot the red line up even higher, right off the chart. She then wrote "OD / Death" beside it. "This is heroin," she explained. I understood what she meant instinctively. I had lived those dramatic highs and lows.

Then she put the red marker down and picked up a green one. This time, she drew a much calmer line—a gentle green wave floating through the graph's centre, never touching the extreme highs or lows. "That's methadone," she said. I understood what Dr. M was saying. The point of methadone was to never feel dopesick or high. If she could get me on the right dose, my life would be like the gentle green line.

In her precise Austrian accent, Dr. M explained why that green line was so important: "When you're in the middle of the graph, you're using your normal, healthy brain," she said. "But when you go to either extreme, the addict's brain takes over." Is this how Dr. M saw me, I thought—as two different people? A normal guy and an addict, both sharing a brain? "The addict's brain is incapable of making good decisions," she said.

I nodded along politely. But I wasn't so sure. There was nothing wrong with my brain when I felt the warm hug of dope. In fact, that's when I felt the most mentally well. On heroin, I liked myself. I was patient, creative and rational. I felt like myself, and wasn't being eaten alive by acidic shame. But at the bottom of the graph I had made all of my worst decisions.

I wanted to get off the graph entirely, and put all drugs behind me. Life at the top of the graph had been good. The undulating up and down was not. But I could never stay at the top. I would have much preferred to be part of the North American Opiate

Medication Initiative prescription heroin study. NAOMI participants got subsidized, daily access to the euphoria I was looking
for. I'd seen posters for NAOMI on the Downtown Eastside. It
looked just like the British system of prescription heroin: they
were giving out legal dope to study participants. But there were
only around one hundred available spaces. And to qualify, you
needed to have first tried—and failed—on methadone. And so,
at least for now, I was stuck with Dr. M.

"But I'm still an addict though, right?" I asked the doc. "It's
just that I'll be addicted to methadone now instead of heroin?"

"No," Dr. M explained. "Physical dependence is different
from addiction. One is addicted to heroin, but dependent on
methadone." This made no sense. Methadone and heroin are
both opioids. After prolonged use, your body will go into withdrawal when either is taken away. It seemed like Dr. M was
lawyering the definitions so methadone came out ahead. This
was a semantic and confusing distinction. Did it just boil down
to "illegal drugs are bad, legal ones are good"?

I opened the *Methadone Maintenance Treatment Client
Handbook*. It said, "People who take methadone as a treatment
for opioid dependence are no more addicts than are people who
take insulin as a treatment for diabetes. Methadone is a medication. Methadone treatment allows you to live a normal life,
work, go to school, or care for your children."

On my way out of the clinic, I grabbed a pamphlet from
the waiting room. It said, "Addiction is about irrationally
choosing the negative consequences from problematic drug
use." I turned the pamphlet over in my hands, thinking about
the phrase "problematic drug use." I had always thought that *I*

was the problem. Not my drug use. But I couldn't deny that my drug use had fucked up my life. I got out my notebook and listed all the problems it had caused me. Dopesickness. Being broke. Police harassment. Lying. Overdoses. And I realized that none of these things would be a problem on methadone, because methadone was legal, subsidized and always the same potency. Yet the exact same thing was true for prescribed heroin in the UK.

It was pointless to parse definitions. Methadone was the only game in town for me. I needed opioids, and Dr. M had them. End of story. I shoved my notebook, the pamphlet and the handbook in my backpack and lit a smoke.

I returned to Dr. M's clinic a few days later. To my relief, she said I was negative for HIV and hep C. And she added that the College of Physicians and Surgeons, which regulated methadone maintenance, had accepted me into the program. I learned later that activists from the demonstration Andy and I attended had been fighting for more spaces in methadone programs. Their advocacy work was probably why I was admitted this time. But now I had another problem. I had to pay for it. My Medical Services Plan card was out of date, which meant the clinic wasn't able to bill the government for my visits. I was also broke and unable to pay their regular monthly fees. The receptionist said they'd let it ride for a few weeks while I sorted things out. But I needed to pay the pharmacy for dispensing the actual medication.

Dr. M wrote me my first script. I'd be starting on forty millilitres of methadone. Dr. M said my dose could be increased in the coming weeks if it wasn't holding me properly. But I didn't want that. A higher dose would take me longer to get off. Worse, if I got kicked out of the program, I'd be more dopesick than if I hadn't come to the clinic in the first place. My methadone would be dispensed daily, which meant I would have to go to the pharmacy every single day. A pharmacist would watch me drink my juice—to make sure I swallowed it all and didn't hold it in my mouth to sell later. The medical system didn't trust people like me, even though it turned out that crooked pharmacists were the ones stealing methadone at scale.

The program required me to organize my life around the medication. It didn't matter if I was sick, if I was dealing with a crisis at work, if there was a blizzard or if there was a funeral that I needed to attend across the country. It was up to me to get my ass to the pharmacy or suffer the consequences. Nearly every methadone patient in Canada and the United States is required to take their methadone under this kind of mandatory surveillance.

"It's part of the treatment," Dr. M told me. "The daily pharmacy trips will put some structure back into your life. Regular visits to the clinic will build a therapeutic relationship between you and I." After all, this wasn't like other kinds of health care.

"You have to *want* to be on this program," she explained frankly. "This is work. Patients have to earn it."

Methadone Flatline

My first step as a new methadone patient was to find a pharmacy. I considered going to one of the sketchier ones—there were plenty in East Van. I knew these places paid methadone patients kickbacks—sometimes a hundred bucks in monthly cash bribes to secure our patronage. Or more. Methadone was big business. The pharmacies collected a dispensing fee every time we took the juice. And they collected an additional fee for watching us drink it. Because so many of us were required to return to the pharmacy every single day, they made thousands a year off each patient. I was broke and desperate. I wanted that monthly kickback. But I also knew that many of the sketchier pharmacies would sell some of their methadone out the back door. And to compensate, they'd water down the juice they dispensed to patients.

Instead, I decided to go to a pharmacy inside a nearby Safeway, where I knew I wouldn't get a kickback, but I hoped the methadone would be legit. I wandered through aisles of produce, bread and canned goods, walking past a family arguing over what kind of cereal to buy. I noticed a security guard behind me, tracking me through the store. At the pharmacy counter, I passed my script to a white-coated technician. She handed back a paper outlining the pharmacy's rules for methadone patients.

"Any instance of deceitful practice or communication, physical or verbal abuse or theft will not be tolerated," the document read. I knew they didn't hand these rule sheets to "normal" customers. But being on methadone meant you were a suspect by default. The pharmacy technician asked me to sign the rule sheet at the bottom, handing me a copy "to retain for my records." She informed me that since my pharma coverage wasn't up to date, I would have to pay fifteen dollars out of pocket, every day, until I got it sorted out. She then measured out forty millilitres of Tang-flavoured methadone into a little plastic cup. I drank the juice down as the technician watched closely, making sure I didn't keep any in my cheeks. It was humiliating. But I was so used to this sort of mistrust and policing, I just went along with it.

As I walked back through Safeway, I noticed the security guard was still following me. I waved. "See ya tomorrow," I said. Then it dawned on me: I had to come back tomorrow. And the next day, and the next day. Methadone was going to be a lot of work. There would be piss tests every time I went to the clinic. Other times they would call me randomly to demand I present myself for urine analysis within twenty-four hours. If I failed to comply, it'd be recorded as a blown test. I knew people who got kicked off the program for too many blown tests. I also had to attend mandatory group counselling once a week.

It was onerous. But I was determined to make this work. I figured the main thing was to manage relationships. I needed to stay on good terms with all of the receptionists, pharmacists, technicians and doctors I'd come across. Especially Dr. M. Whenever I walked into her clinic, I'd code-switch to a persona of cheerful institutional compliance—a useful mask I'd donned around bosses, cops, prison guards and landlords. The key was not only to follow their rules, but to appear to like them. I wanted authority figures to think I agreed with the logic behind their requirements. I wanted to become a frictionless surface, where no conflict could stick to me.

My mandatory support group met in a room in the clinic with information posters on the wall about hep C, diet and exercise. People took their chairs and chatted with each other. This was my first session, but the eight other attendees seemed to already know each other. People wore a mix of work clothes and athletic gear. A woman named Danielle was the facilitator. She wore a thick turtleneck sweater and chunky jewellery. There was no coffee. Danielle got the meeting started.

I wondered if any of my fellow clinic patients would blab to the world that I was here. There were a few journalists in the city who were always looking for ways to take down activists, and I worried I would discredit the organizations I worked with if my drug use was made public. I was trying to hide my heroin use from people in my life. But I was even more determined to keep people from knowing I was on methadone. Because being on methadone meant—beyond a shadow of doubt—that I was an addict. I wasn't a rebel, a rock star, or an outlaw, just a loser with a drug problem.

"Hi, everyone," one of the participants said in a gravelly smoker's voice. Crystal had short, spiky black hair and wore a denim jacket with the sleeves ripped off. I noticed she was sitting slightly doubled over, holding her stomach. "I haven't pooped in two weeks," she volunteered. It was a brilliant way to break the ice. The group erupted in sympathy, sharing stories and suggesting cures to commiserate. Isaac told us he was only shitting rabbit pellets. Roy turned to Crystal and said, "I shit a baseball and broke my ass. I got an anal fissure." Everyone laughed until Danielle, the facilitator, called us back to order. I didn't volunteer any similar information, but the truth was that I was backed up too. All opioids had that effect on you, especially methadone. "All this talk is making me think I'm gonna crap my pants," Crystal said, and she excused herself. Everyone giggled awkwardly as she left the room.

Danielle handed out an info sheet called "Constipation Management." It instructed us to drink eight glasses of water each day. We were also supposed to eat All-Bran, exercise regularly and use stool softeners and Metamucil if necessary. "Develop good bowel habits," the info sheet said. "Get into a routine and ensure you have some quiet time in the bathroom after breakfast." Since I didn't sleep properly or eat regular meals, this would require an overhaul of my whole life. "Quiet time in the bathroom" was to be another part of my new, super-uncool methadone career.

I was going to have to step up my dental care as well. I learned that methadone gives you dry mouth, robbing you of saliva. And this can cause tooth decay. Jeff had lost his teeth after contracting a superbug in the hospital. And he warned me to hang on to mine as long as I could. I got an electric toothbrush and attacked my teeth for a couple of minutes, morning and night.

At the next clinic support group meeting, Crystal's voice was subdued. She told us her boyfriend had stolen her AA chip. Crystal wasn't telling those at her AA meeting she was on the methadone program because nearly every twelve-step group regarded taking methadone to be active drug use. But she was proud of her clean time from alcohol, and that chip meant a lot to her. Crystal cried and told us that her boyfriend often beat her up and stole from her. "Why do I always end up with these guys?" she sniffled.

Danielle asked each of us to go home and write a letter to Crystal for the next session expressing what we liked about her. I hardly knew Crystal and felt a bit awkward about the assignment. But I also felt bad for her situation with her boyfriend, so I did the best I could. At the next session, I realized that I was the only one who had completed the assignment. I passed my folded letter to Crystal and she accepted it, slowly unfolding the page. We all listened as she read my words aloud. I felt embarrassed, but after just a few seconds, tears were streaking her mascara. "I love it," Crystal said. "Nobody's ever written something like this for me before." I felt a little flash of pride. But the mood abruptly soured when Crystal added, "I can't keep this." She held the letter out for me to take back. "My boyfriend goes through my stuff and if he finds it, he'll kill me."

I still didn't trust the juice to hold me. I was on the edge of dopesickness all the time, so I topped up with heroin. I soon learned that most of the people in the support group were doing the same thing. Some patients would even go score together after group. But we knew better than to be honest about that in front of Danielle because we knew we could always be kicked off the program for any kind of disobedience. This threat was an intentional part of the program's design. It was there to motivate us to settle for the numbness of methadone—and not to chase the euphoria that led us to get wired in the first place.

I had been on the program for about six months when the government confirmed that my health coverage was finally fixed and that my income was sufficiently low to qualify for subsidized pharmacare. This relieved some of the financial pressure. I still had to pay the clinic fees—about sixty dollars per month—but I didn't have to hand over $15 at the pharmacy every day. It had been brutal keeping up with those payments, and I had missed several doses because of it.

One time I missed the pharmacy and didn't go back for six days. The pharmacy cancelled my prescription, and I had to go back to Dr. M and explain myself. She restarted me at a lower dose. Then I missed the pharmacy for another four days. I repeated this pattern several times, unconsciously reaching for the relief heroin used to bring me before methadone. I was stuck in a purgatory between the drugs. Eventually my dose got to 130 millilitres. That number seemed big. One day I wanted to get off this stuff, but I knew that wasn't going to be anytime soon. The higher up I went, the harder it would be to get back down. And, if I got cut off, I'd have to replace the methadone equivalent with street dope. Out of curiosity, I asked Dr. M how fast I could get off the juice. She warned that she hadn't seen much success from people rushing the process. She advised me to stabilize first before thinking about tapers.

In the waiting room, support group and pharmacy, I'd talk to other methadone patients. We'd compare the number of millilitres we were on and our plans to get off methadone soon. We counted millilitres like twelve-steppers counted clean time, congratulating each other when we shaved our dose down a little, commiserating when it crept up.

Rebecca was part of the clinic support group. She was rushing to get herself off methadone before she got married. "I'm gonna be clean when I walk down that aisle," she said, showing us her engagement ring. "I don't want Daddy giving away a dirty daughter." Her wedding was a few months away, and we were all rooting for her. After all, this is what success looked like to us. We were all dirty daughters. And many of us wanted to show our dads that we could get clean.

An older guy with short grey hair stopped coming to group. I bumped into him on the street and asked what was up. "I just can't fucking stand it," he said. He didn't like all the surveillance, piss tests and pharmacists watching you. "I'm not a child," he said, "I gotta work. I can't get to the pharmacy every morning."

After a year and a half on the methadone program, I was still pissing hot every time. But I wasn't feeling the dope. The heroin was fighting with the methadone, and the methadone was winning. Methadone was stealthier than any dope I'd known. It was tactical, crafty, nimble, worming its way in and sitting on the opioid receptors in my brain, where it acted like a security guard. If any heroin molecules floated past, the methadone said, "Keep moving, we're full up here."

It seemed like lots of us at the clinic were having this problem. We were less sick than we used to be, but we were missing the buzz. I tried smoking rock. I tried benzodiazepines. I even smoked weed—a drug that I'd come to think of as weak and pedestrian. But nothing replaced the relief that heroin gave me. Dilaudid came the closest. Sue was my regular Dilly dealer. She lived at the Hazelwood Hotel and sold Dilly 8s (eight-milligram opioid pills) for ten bucks a pop. She'd give me a discount when I bought in bulk, which I always did. Because, on methadone, I needed a handful of Dillies to get high.

Dr. M could see all of this in my piss tests. She said that I seemed "ambivalent" about the program, and that I was showing little commitment. She told me people in my situation usually drop out. And—as a last-ditch effort—she registered me in an addiction day-treatment program. I looked at the Family Services of Greater Vancouver brochure. The cover showed a seagull soaring in a blue sky. The brochure said I could take either a three-week program called "Healing and the Art of Recovery" or a five-week program called "Recovery Skills." But I knew I'd be asked to open up—to share the dark stories that motivated my drug use. I had spent a lifetime avoiding my demons, and I wasn't ready to confront them. So I never showed up to the intake appointment. It felt like just a matter of time before Dr. M had had enough of me.

But then things changed. I don't know exactly when it happened. It was gradual. But at some point, I started to trust methadone. Before I was on the program, outrunning dope-sickness had been my full-time job. It was exhausting. Now, I'd gone months on end without feeling sick. At first I didn't do much with my newfound time and energy. I just sat at home, listening to music. I felt a big greyness, a broad-spectrum lack. I had forgotten how to live a normal life. But eventually I realized I could overcome the inertia. I just had to remember the moves.

It started small. Once a week I'd take the bus to visit my uncle Johnny. The receptionist at Johnny's long-term care home would give me taxi vouchers so that I could take him to his oncology appointments. After seeing the doctor, Uncle Johnny and I would eat lunch in the cancer centre cafeteria. He always ate the same thing: a turkey sandwich, which he'd wash down with a small carton of 2 per cent milk. We chatted about working at mines. Johnny had been the butcher at the Bralorne Mine, west of Lillooet, BC. It felt good to be useful to someone in the family.

I also took care of Paige. Sometimes my sister would pass Paige out the window of their ground-floor East Van apartment and we'd play on the grass. When my sister was out, I babysat. Paige would point to a couple of places on my guitar, and we'd write and sing little songs together about whatever she wanted. We wrote one about the moon and another about her mom. She'd fall asleep in my lap, and when Gill came home, I'd often be asleep too. I gave Paige musical instruments for every birthday and Christmas. When Paige started school, I went to parent-teacher night.

Jeff and I met up for breakfast at the Ovaltine Cafe at least once a week. I had been nagging him to try methadone since I got on the program. He was suspicious of anything to do with the medical system. Eventually he did, and his doctor also prescribed slow-release oral morphine for his pain. That combination was really working out for him.

After years of failure, I was thirsty for success. I started to develop a pattern with the methadone. I drank my juice every morning. I even bought a little extra off the street to build up a small emergency stockpile. That way, if the pharmacy had a shortage, I'd be able to stay on track. I started to use other drugs less and less. I still needed to get properly high when I felt like shit. But I no longer felt like shit every day. I was learning to make peace with the green centreline. It wasn't terrible being in the middle. And I could tell Dr. M was impressed with my progress.

Dr. M stopped writing "daily witness" on my scripts. Instead, I got carries. I was beaming with pride on the way to the pharmacy. It felt like I had robbed the place when I walked out with a paper bag containing a half-dozen amber bottles of methadone—each with a sticker that said "poison." I wouldn't have to come back to the pharmacy for a full week. I could just pull a bottle from my fridge in the morning. My liquid hand-cuffs felt looser.

In 2004, I started an office job. I was analyzing the social and environmental impacts of industrial development in BC. In the beige cubicle farm, I felt like I had a giant "addict" sign on my forehead. I imagined a hundred different ways my bosses and colleagues might discover I had a habit. But it never happened. Turns out, I was like millions of other drug users who go to work every day, their co-workers and family none the wiser.

When my three-month contract came to an end, my position was extended for another year. I became a union member and got extended health benefits. I did my job and was pretty good at it, making strong relationships with the people I worked alongside.

Having a stable job meant that I was finally able to pay down my debts. I cleared up my unpaid fees at the methadone clinic. I settled up with Lee and the other dealers I owed money to around town. And I paid back all of the friends who'd ever helped me out. I no longer needed to worry about eviction notices. I bought myself a new biker jacket.

After a couple years, I became a shop steward with my union, the Canadian Association of Professional Employees. Then I was elected president of Local 301. I met a woman named April. She worked near where I worked, and we started dating. It was important to me to date someone who didn't use hard drugs.

Over bacon and eggs, Jeff told me he had also met someone. He moved out of the Balmoral Hotel, out of the Downtown Eastside and in with her—into a big green apartment building near the beach, with a view of Burrard Inlet and the North Shore Mountains. The methadone, morphine prescription and the girlfriend seemed like the right combination for Jeff. He told me proudly that he'd stopped using heroin and was only using rock—in addition to his prescriptions. He laughed and said, "I'm retired." We were both amazed that a legal supervised injection site had been opened on the 100 block of East Hastings and had managed to stay open, despite opposition from pundits and police. We clinked coffee mugs. This seemed like a win.

Fewer sirens were screaming by. The newspapers had moved on from the public health crises of the 1990s. It seemed like that terrible era of mass death was wrapping up—or at least deaths from overdoses and HIV transmission were returning to lower levels. Years later, Dr. John Blatherwick, then chair of the Vancouver/Richmond Health Board, explained to local journalist Travis Lupick, "It was simply a numbers game . . . the epidemic just burned itself out." It was a grim conclusion. There weren't enough of us left to keep the body count so high. It was hard to believe it was over.

On the bus, I saw that I had a voicemail message. I played it back. It was a child's voice saying, "Big monkey, little monkey. Big monkey, little monkey. Big monkey, little monkey." Paige was three and had apparently just figured out how to use the phone. I had no idea what she was talking about, but I played the message back again and again, laughing each time. Paige was a little bit of light in my life. I loved her.

My methadone support group was working out too. "Excellent participation," Danielle wrote on my attendance card. "Great addition to the group." Danielle said she was impressed at how confident I was becoming. She said it seemed like I had "learned to deal with things as they arise and not let them get out of control." It was good to get positive feedback. Around that time, the clinic stopped offering counselling.

I had made peace with methadone. I was no longer in a hurry to wean myself off. At least not anytime soon. *If it ain't broke, don't fix it,* I thought. But I did want to stop using other drugs.

Defects of Character

We were doomed from the start. April was a glamorous party girl, and I was a boring office worker. She was a tattoo artist who worked out of a studio near my building and was into alternative dance music, while I still liked old-school punk rock. April didn't have a dope habit like me. But after a night at the bar, or dancing at a club, I'd often have to hold her up as we staggered down the street. I got messed up, but I didn't really party. My use was private and personal. April was a weekend warrior who sometimes waged war on weekdays too. I couldn't keep up.

April and I had been dating for a little over a year. I still had my carries. But I didn't feel much pride anymore. I was using Dilaudid and morphine more often. At first I'd been able to hide it from April, using when she wasn't around. But eventually she figured out what was going on and suggested that we go to a twelve-step meeting.

I'd been down this road plenty of times. Over the years, I'd gone to NA meetings in Ottawa, Prince Rupert, Terrace and Fort St. John. I once even tried to go to a meeting aboard a ship. I tried to act eager about the idea, but I knew that twelve-step wasn't really my bag. And I also knew that you were supposed to go to those meetings because *you* had a desire to stop using. Not because your girlfriend wanted you to. By "Higher Power," the Big Book didn't mean your old lady.

But another part of me was open to the idea. My life was a bit more stable now than it was the last time I'd tried the program. Maybe the combination of methadone and twelve-step would work. Maybe it'd be different this time. Fuck it. It was a Hail Mary. If I didn't try something, I knew I'd be alone again in no time.

I imagined the tasks. Writing out lists of my moral defects, the people I'd wronged and to whom I'd need to make amends. My parents, who I'd caused worry, embarrassment and disappointment. My late grandfather, who I had been close to until I was around ten—a relationship I let grow distant. Relationships, like with Nina, where I chose heroin over my partner. Former bandmates. Taxpayers. People who tried to help me. People who I should have helped. Society at large.

While April fixed her makeup, I picked up my dog-eared, large-print copy of the Narcotics Anonymous Basic Text. I'd got it at a group that met in the basement of St. James' Anglican Church on the Downtown Eastside. Sad documentation of previous failed attempts. As I went to shove the book in my backpack, it flopped open to a passage: "Addicts are self-centered, angry, frightened and lonely people . . . dishonest, self-seeking and often institutionalized." It was like a slap in the face. What if that was me? The text gnawed at my self-esteem.

On the bus to the meeting, April and I sat together in silence. I could feel us drifting apart. It wasn't just drugs, it was activism too. I was part of a group called the Olympic Resistance

Network. Vancouver was going to host the Olympic Winter Games the following year. Our group was concerned about the skyrocketing rents, evictions and increased police harassment that came with the Games. But the Olympics were popular, and the city felt like it was caught in one long pep rally. Every week we had meetings and teach-ins. April wasn't interested. I didn't blame her.

The police had formed a new combined unit, fat with Olympics dollars. They were monitoring a dozen activists, including me. Three cops questioned me one day as I left a debate at City Hall. Another time, as I was leaving work, two plainclothes cops followed me, asking questions. "What are your plans during the Games?" the older one inquired politely. "It would be too bad if someone got the wrong idea about you and thought you were a threat," the young, muscular one said, menacingly. "It would be a shame if we had to talk to your boss." Other cops knocked on my neighbours' doors, asking them about me. I didn't want the police to find out I was a dope-fiend going to NA—but they probably knew already.

April and I got off the bus and joined a knot of smokers on Sophia Street outside the Recovery Club. There were a couple nods of recognition. I didn't know if people recognized me personally or just recognized what I was here for. Dressed in hoodies and leather jackets, jeans and Adidas trackies, they chatted quietly. Some drank coffee from Styrofoam cups. It was mostly beards, stubble and ball caps. Besides April, there was only one other woman there. She was rummaging around her handbag and announced that the next meeting started in five minutes.

"Hey, man," an old-school biker said to me brightly. He had the confident swagger of a veteran. I could tell he was a seasoned practitioner of the sober arts. "Back again, eh?" he laughed. Some of the others laughed too. It was a common icebreaker. I wasn't sure if I'd ever met this guy before, but I guess I had "back again" written all over my face.

Pre-meeting smokes were my favourite part. I'd stand on the sidewalk or sit on a picnic table, listening to people's war stories and just enjoying the camaraderie. Nobody was out to boss you around. Nobody was trying to make money off you. Most of the people were earnest, trying to make an honest change. It was a real fellowship. I liked the people here, mostly. But my creep radar pinged as this one older guy moved in beside April.

"How long have you been in the program?" he asked her, his voice light and supplicating.

"This is my first meeting," she said.

"That's great. I've got five years," he said, waving a black key fob. "Do you have a sponsor yet?" *Okay*, I thought, *here we go.* "We should exchange numbers," he continued, taking a step closer to April. He lowered his voice. "You're going to need plenty of support." April took a step toward me, trying to indicate we were together. She looked uncomfortable.

I could tell right away this guy was working on his "thirteenth step." There always seemed to be some creepy fellowship veteran dude trying to take a younger woman under his wing. April looped her arm through mine. The creepy guy got the message and began chatting to the woman with the handbag instead.

There were people I needed to avoid at the meeting as well. The thirteenth-steppers had zero interest in me, but the sober evangelists, with their new-convert zeal, always seemed to gravitate to me. I guess I radiated "addict who still suffers." The sober evangelists had found something that worked for them, which made them absolutely certain that it would work for me too. It was impossible to convince them otherwise—even though the majority of people who try twelve-step don't stay sober.

Don't get me wrong. I wanted to make the program work. But I couldn't help feeling turned off by the guys who called themselves "dopeless hope-fiends." I was much more comfortable sitting with the skeptics at the back of the class. The guys who'd whisper "Don't relapse without me" after the meeting.

The biker veteran and I stubbed out our smokes. *Funny how this is okay*, I thought to myself. Cigarettes aren't just permitted in NA—they're practically a requirement, even though smoking is addictive and kills way more people than drugs. "Nobody ever robbed a bank to buy darts," the biker said to me, like he'd read my mind. Then he added, in his "of service" voice, "When we look for loopholes in the program, like a lawyer, we're just looking for an easy way out. It's just your addiction talking, bud." I remembered Dr. M telling me how the "addict's brain" can't make good choices.

It was time to go up to the meeting. The biker turned to head back inside, gesturing for April and me to follow. "Let's get at 'er." Upstairs, down the hall and inside the meeting room, chairs were set out and leaflets arranged at the front on a trapezoidal table like they had at my elementary school. April and I took our seats. I looked down at the familiar tile floor, patterned in a checkerboard of grey and darker grey. Fluorescent lights gave everything a monochrome wash, including the people. The biker sat at the front, behind the table. "Welcome! My name is Ben and I am an addict."

"Hi, Ben," most of the room said in unison.

"Is this anyone's first meeting?" Ben asked. April put up her hand.

"Is anyone coming back?" Ben meant was there anyone who had relapsed and was returning to start over. Lots of hands shot up. Including mine.

Most of the people here were twelve-step veterans. Most had been to an outpatient program, like Dr. M had suggested I go to, or had white-knuckled it in Vancouver Detox, which was located in the city's old dog pound. There were also plenty of residential recovery veterans from places across the province. Programs raved about their "tough love" approach to addiction, which basically meant they'd force you to be totally abstinent. Some places allowed Suboxone, an opioid substitution treatment like methadone, but they'd put you on a fast taper off of it.

The government subsidized many such places without requiring them to show any evidence of success. They never had to declare how many clients they'd kicked out versus how many actually graduated from their programs. And that meant, if you slipped up, they were more than happy to kick you to the curb. The government also didn't regulate what kind of "psychosocial programming" these facilities had to provide, or what kind of training their counsellors were required to have. And so most of the places opted for amateur staff and sent their clients to the cheapest programming possible. Residents had to haul their asses to an unaffiliated twelve-step program nearby. Like this one.

Many drug users had also been unlucky enough to wind up in one of the nameless small private recovery houses littered across Surrey. Here, they didn't even pretend to care about "recovery." The residents were often placed there as a condition of their release from prison. They lived under the thumb of the house's owner—often just a dealer or gangster looking to steal their methadone kickbacks. Anyone who's lived in one of these places will tell you there's a better chance you'll die in a fire than get sober there. These shitty houses in Surrey don't have a monopoly on this kind of exploitation. According to allegations in a 2021 *Prince George Citizen* article, the Baldy Hughes Therapeutic Community forced clients to work the phones on behalf of a provincial politician. The facility denied it. But if you're in the life, you know that the recovery scene is full of these kinds of rackets.

None of this is ever mentioned by the endless carousel of politicians who promise to fix Canada's drug problem. In every city, you can find some asshole standing on a soapbox, yapping about all the money that goes toward saving people from overdoses, HIV and hep C. Instead, they'll say, we should put that money toward "recovery." They never specify what that means. We just need more "beds." These beds should be *somewhere* where *someone* is doing *something*—but those details don't matter. The point is really just to make us go away. To put us out of sight.

In Vancouver, there's often talk of reopening Riverview, the old mental hospital. Maybe the drug users could be disappeared there? Sometimes the politicians say that we should give more power to cops. Maybe the cops should be given the right to drag drug users off to a recovery facility against their will? Maybe we should be confined in there? And in many jurisdictions, they've done just that: they've passed laws making involuntary treatment an everyday response to drug use, even though mountains of evidence show that people do not succeed at recovery when they're forced or coerced into it.

In spite of all of these political talking points, BC still doesn't have a decent *voluntary*, evidence-based recovery system. In Vancouver, you have to get on a waiting list just to get into detox. After that, you're put on another waiting list—often months long—before you can graduate to one of the scandal-ridden, under-regulated, private for-profit recovery houses. If you can't get a government-subsidized spot, which are limited, it can cost between $9,000 and $15,000 per month to stay in these places. Families remortgage their homes to send their kids there. And some continue to pay off the recovery house after their kid has overdosed and died. Which is not unlikely—because people tend to relapse right after getting kicked out of recovery, this time with a lowered tolerance and disrupted connections to trusted dealers.

"Well, keep coming back," Ben said from the front. "We ask that no drugs or drug paraphernalia be on your person at the meeting." He asked someone to pass out books. Only a few people, like me, had brought our own.

We opened our Basic Texts, and Ben started to nominate readers around the room. We each took turns reading the steps out loud. Some stumbled with the words. As people read, I noticed that the steps were all in past tense. As if we'd completed them already. Someone read: "We admitted that we were power-less, with unmanageable lives. We admitted that only God could fix us—if we let him."

"We made a searching and fearless moral inventory of ourselves."

"We told someone—in detail—the nature of our wrongs."

"We let God remove our defects of character and short-comings."

"We made lists of everybody we'd harmed and asked them to forgive us."

"We had a spiritual awakening."

And, finally, "We had to carry the message to the addict who still suffers."

At the end of the steps, you have to start working them again but I'd never really gotten past the first step before. I already felt powerless, I didn't feel comfortable about the God or spiritual awakening stuff, and I knew I didn't have a defective character. Ben could see how daunting this all sounded. "There's no work in the first three steps. Only acceptance and understanding," he said. "Then comes the work." Polite laughter. "Now you're gonna read from the Basic Text, okay?" he said to April.

April beamed and sat up a little straighter. "Who is an addict?" she said, looking around the room. Then she looked down at the book in her hands. "Most of us do not have to think twice about this question. WE KNOW!" There were nods. Someone said, "Hell yeah, we do!"

April continued reading: "We lived to use and used to live. We are people in the grip of a continuing and progressive illness whose ends are always the same: jails, institutions and death."

The room was silent, listening intently. Even those who'd obviously heard this passage before nodded along.

"We did not choose to become addicts," April read. "We suffer from a disease. Our disease isolated us from people. Hostile, resentful, self-centered and self-seeking, we cut ourselves off from the outside world. . . . We lied, stole, cheated and sold ourselves. We had to have drugs, regardless of the cost. Failure and fear began to invade our lives." It seemed to me that a lot of this stealing and lying was about money, not disease. The illicit market made drugs needlessly expensive. And we wound up in jail because drugs are illegal, not because we were broken. I didn't see how it helped to constantly repeat that we were terrible people. I knew I wasn't all those things. But the Recovery Club was no place to commit sociology.

There was a little discussion of the meaning of all that. A guy named Chris said, "All decisions I made, I did so out of fear." And people mumbled their agreement. April listened, leaned forward, nodding along. She was here to support me, but she seemed to be getting something out of this anyway.

April nudged me when the chair asked if anyone else wanted to share. But I couldn't explain what was wrong with me and why I needed dope. I couldn't tell them that dope was where I turned for acceptance and relief. My truth was heresy: heroin was my Higher Power. In these rooms, I knew my story would sound like a rationalization. So I said nothing.

Up at the front, Ben said, "Remember HALTS. Don't let yourself get too hungry, angry, lonely, tired . . . or serious!" He stood up and squared his shoulders, "This group recognizes clean time by handing out key tags. If you have one coming to you, please come up and get it." Slowly, the attendees approached the front as if this were an altar call. "Anyone got a month? Thirty days clean and serene?" Ben asked. The woman with the handbag accepted an orange key tag. Next Ben called for people with sixty days. They got a green one. When Ben called for the people who'd cleared ninety days, two stood up. There was a smattering of applause as they accepted their red tags. The applause got louder as the time increased: blue tags for six months, yellow tags for nine months, and a glow-in-the-dark tag for one year. People who had been clean for multiple years got the ultimate prize—black tags. I bet Ben had one of those himself.

"All those with the desire to stay clean today, give yourself a hand. You are the most important people in the room." Some people clapped at me. I couldn't imagine a lifetime of sobriety. They may as well have asked me to fly to Yellowknife by flapping my arms. "Come and collect your key tags."

April nudged me to go up. Ben gave me a white plastic key fob on a metal ring. I turned the key fob over in my hand. It had the NA logo and "welcome" printed on one side. On the other it said "Just for today" in gold letters. I already had a few at home. Ben looked me in the eye and said, "Keep coming back, brother."

The key fob was a reminder of the one requirement of membership: the desire to stop using drugs—including methadone. But I wanted to stay on methadone—for now—and quit everything else. That didn't count as sobriety here. The NA Basic Text said, "We are allergic to drugs. It would be insane to go back to the source of our allergy. Medicine cannot 'cure' our illness." NA Bulletin #29 was even more direct. "Our program approaches recovery from addiction through abstinence, cautioning against the substitution of one drug for another." There was no nuance to all the Basic Text readings. It was a binary, absolutist approach to recovery—all or nothing. You were clean or dirty. You were saved or a sinner.

I didn't want to lie to Ben and the other volunteers who ran this meeting. They weren't paid to be here. They were drug users like me, just trying to get well. But then again, the creator of the twelve-step system, Bill W., wasn't totally abstinent himself when he dreamed up this regime. In 1934, while in hospital, Bill W. claimed to have seen a white light that cured his alcoholism in one hot flash. The thing is, he was being treated at the time with belladonna, a hallucinogenic plant. It seemed that even the founder needed a little psychoactive assistance.

Ben had us bow our heads in a moment of silence "for the addict who still suffers." Then we huddled for a group hug. April got right in there. The creepy guy snuck in beside her, so I joined in too. Arm in arm, in a big circle, we all recited the Serenity Prayer. "God, grant me the serenity to accept the things I cannot change, the courage to change the things I can, and the wisdom to know the difference." I mumbled along, conscious of a lifetime spent fighting things I couldn't change. As the hug dispersed, the handbag woman approached Ben with a piece of paper. Without a word, he signed it, proving she'd been at the meeting. She had been ordered by the court to attend NA.

Outside, a couple of the more seasoned members talked about their lives. I could tell by the cadences that these stories had been told again and again. And I already knew how they went. You start with a cinematic snapshot of your past life in all of its debauched chaos. The time you pissed in the back seat of a cop car. Hold for laughs. Then comes the pivot to a great loss. The people you loved that you can't get back. The wife left. She took the kids. This is the part of the story that'll break the listener's heart. You aren't the victim here. All that suffering is your fault. Then comes the turn—a sinner struck by a revelation from the Lord. You're saved. A new man—the comeback kid, born again. The horror of your old life only testifies to the glory of your new life. Of course, the redemption story arc always needs a bit of editing. Dozens of relapses don't really fit into this narrative.

Twelve-steppers know how to spin a yarn. I've often thought that this is probably the most effective part of the program: twelve-step gives you a community and it teaches you to tell a new story about yourself. One where you're not a piece of shit anymore. Waggling a black key fob, one guy said, "Five hundred and twelve days clean!" I was genuinely impressed. Five hundred and twelve days was an impossibly long time, geologic even.

I wished that I could chime in with my own redemption story. But I didn't see any way of rearranging the sea of depressing shit that I'd done—and that had been done to me—into any kind of uplifting sequence. So I stood in silence, listening to everyone else's story. Before taking off, Ben gave me a list of phone numbers of other members. "Reach out if you're feeling weak," he said, with genuine care. He waved goodbye to April and me and pointed at the list in my hand. "Use it," he said.

Fat chance, I thought.

Another Overload

'm floating somewhere, way far out. There's a radio on, miles away. "Accident mid-span on Ironworkers Bridge . . ." I don't know where I am. A song comes on with a smooth, melancholic voice that croons about a lonely lineman, endlessly searching an electrical grid for overloaded circuits. The wires sing to him. This mellow ballad isn't the kind of music I usually like, but it's so beautiful, I could cry. What's this song called again?

Am I sleeping? I try to wake up, to focus on something—but nothing's coming through. It's weird. There's another sound somewhere, low in the mix. Some kind of wailing. I need to pay attention to this. It's fading up. *That's a siren.* I wonder who it's for.

Shit. Wait a minute. What's going on? I think it's an ambulance. A lazy butterfly notion flutters into my skull: Is that siren for me?

I think the song is called "Wichita Lineman." Where's my notebook? I need to write that down before I forget. I can't remember anything. Where am I? What time is it?

The siren gets louder and louder. It hurts. Until all of a sudden, it stops.

Shadowy outlines of strangers move around me. What are they doing? Their movements are deliberate, calm and professional. This is just a really deep nod.

"I'm okay," I mumble.

I want to go deeper. Let me go. Let me fall into the deep heart of it. Let me sit on the ocean floor. Let me go to that underwater nothing place. I'm not feeling guilty or regretful. I don't have to hide from anybody. I'm not disappointing anybody. It's all finally over. Don't wake me up.

I feel a warm sleeping bag around me. I hear Zippo mumbling in his sleep: "Death is only a heartbeat away." It's not a warning, it's meant to be comforting. This can all be over. I can be with Nick. With Grandpa.

I feel the warm relief of the midnight sun on my face. I lie on the rocks and look into the dome of the sky. Blue fading into violet into blue-black indigo. I hear the loon's note-bending call echo across the giant quiet at the top of the world. I hold on to the rock. Rough, flat and gritty. If I let go, I'll fall straight up, into space, into the black forever, and I'll be gone.

"What did he take?" It's a professional-sounding voice. Business-like, not frantic.

"I don't know," a familiar woman's voice answers. She's not nearly as calm.

It's a good question. What did I take? I have no fucking idea. Did I take my methadone this morning? Probably. And some other opioids. And benzodiazepines. I can't be sure. I should tell them, but I can't get the words out. Why am I cold? No . . . I'm not ready. I don't wanna go.

My autopsy will read: "Albino reptile, dead before forty. No moustache. Collapsed veins. Defects of character." I'm moving smoothly, someone's pushing me. I'm in a wheelchair now. Something is clipped to my finger.

I concentrate on breathing. Deep breath in. Deep breath out.

As the breath returns to me, I feel a little better. This isn't the end. I'll be okay. And as soon as I realize that, my defences go up. *I can't let them put me in that ambulance.* I know the paramedics will Narcan me. And once they knock the opioids out of me, the warm dream will be gone all at once. I'll be in a precipitated withdrawal—shitting and puking alone—sicker than I've ever been.

"I'm fine," I say, more clearly than last time.

The paramedic is holding my arm. I need to get him off me.

Inhale. Gotta make sure my brain is getting enough oxygen.

I stand up and start walking, but my legs are like noodles. "Leaving against medical advice . . . there's nothing we can do . . ." I hear the business-like voice behind me.

Exhale.

The sky is a warm yellow haze. It's golden hour. Most of the day has slipped by without me noticing. Crows are cawing somewhere.

"Garth!"

April is looming over me. Her black hair is hanging down. Her forehead is crinkled in worry and irritation. I smell chow mein. April bought Chinese food.

"Eat this," she says. I take a bite, but then I drift away again. She wakes me and makes me eat again. She does this over and over.

"I'm fine," I say.

"Okay, okay," April says. "Just stay awake."

I try to piece the day together, but I can only remember a few minutes out of the last six hours. She explains slowly. Again and again. I finally understand what happened to me. I overdosed. I'd been here a half-dozen times before, but this is the worst one by far. The closest to death.

"You're so fucked up." April is pissed off. Or maybe she's just worried.

I'm grateful for her support—for taking me to NA and for whatever she did to keep me alive this day. But she'd be better off without me. Maybe everyone would be.

PART 3
GETTING
ORGANIZED

Give Up the Ghost

sauntered down the block, humming to myself. Last year's overdose had scared me. I'd managed to survive on methadone and nothing else since then. I was feeling pretty good. I must have looked a little weird in my combat boots and bathrobe, but I didn't care. It was the weekend, and I had a date with someone I really liked.

Lisa was from the riot grrrl punk scene in Vancouver. We'd been dating for a couple of months and I'd managed to show her my best side, so far. It seemed like she was into me too. We had run into each other at a few gigs, and we were both at the APEC protests when cops pepper-sprayed the crowd. Lisa told me that she'd recently lived in the former Yugoslavia, where she'd been making freelance radio documentaries for the CBC. She'd moved back to Vancouver and started teaching a history course at a local college. She was smart, cute and funny as hell.

Today I was planning on making Lisa brunch at my place. She'd bike over in about an hour. But first, I needed to make a quick trip to the pharmacy. I was looking forward to chatting with the guy who'd been dispensing my methadone for years. We'd developed a nice rapport. *I might even tell him about Lisa,*

I thought. But when I got to the pharmacy, I realized someone new was behind the counter.

"Hi. Prescription for Mullins, please?" I said in a job interview voice. "I'm here to pick up my methadone."

"Okay . . ." the new pharmacist said in a neutral tone. He punched at his keyboard and squinted at the screen in front of him. "Hmm . . ." he said from behind the Plexiglas. "I don't see anything here."

"It should be there," I said, trying not to get ahead of myself. "I come here every week."

"I don't see it," the pharmacist shrugged. "Maybe your doctor forgot to fax it to us?"

"Can you check again?" I asked, my politeness straining a little.

"Sorry about that," the pharmacist said in a tone that made clear our conversation was done. "You'll have to talk to your doctor."

A wave of panic crashed over me. I had used up all my emergency stockpile of methadone, and the clinic wouldn't be open until Monday. I was now doomed to days of dopesickness, just when Lisa and I were getting to know each other. What was I going to do?

Maybe I can reach this guy on some kind of human level. Maybe I can tell him about my overdose last year. Maybe I can tell him about how hard I've been working to avoid dope. Maybe he'll cut me some slack. But then I thought better. No pharmacist in the world is going to believe a dopefiend without a prescription. The clock had already started. Pleading my case would just waste valuable time.

As I rushed home, I called Jeff. I told him the situation and said I'd catch a bus as soon as I could and meet him on Pill Corner. Jeff said he'd help me score something. Methadone was my first choice. But if I couldn't find juice, I'd settle for Dilaudid. Or morphine, or Percocet, or Oxy. It didn't really matter. Just not heroin. That would be my last resort.

At my apartment, I auditioned some excuses in my head to cancel my date with Lisa. Lisa didn't do dope, and I figured she wouldn't understand any of this. She knew me as a guy with a job, a clean apartment and a good coffee maker. But I was already sweating. I checked my watch. *Fuck*. Lisa would be here any minute.

Then the phone rang. It was too late. Lisa was already buzzing up. I hung up my bathrobe, pulled on some clothes and ran down the stairs to meet her at the front door.

Act calm, I told myself.

"Hi! How are you?" I said way too fast. *That wasn't calm at all.*

I needed to feed Lisa some line of bullshit. It didn't matter what it was. "I got called into work." "I have to go help a friend with something." Whatever. *Just shake her off.* This was the kind of lie I was used to delivering without hesitation. But for some reason, nothing was coming to me.

"I'm sorry if this sounds weird," I said, barely believing what I was about to do. "The pharmacy wouldn't give me my methadone and . . ." I checked Lisa's face. She wasn't recoiling yet.

" . . . I need to go obtain an alternative."

Lisa was nodding along. *Why is she cool with this?* I wondered.

I explained the situation as rosily as I could. This was really bad timing. I'm normally not like this at all. But I was already starting to feel rough. If I didn't act fast I'd soon be a total mess.

"We can still hang out in a few days if you want!" I told her.

"Where do we have to go?" Lisa asked. She was ignoring my attempts to brush her off.

"*Please* don't come with me," I said.

"You don't look so good. I'm worried about you," she said. "If you don't let me get on that bus with you, I'll just follow on my bike."

"Okay," I replied. This was such a bad idea.

Lisa and I waited together until the bus finally arrived. It felt like hours. I tried to hide how sick I was feeling as our bus drove to the Downtown Eastside.

When we arrived a few minutes later, Jeff was waiting. I breathed a sigh of relief. I knew he'd take over now. "No one's selling methadone today," he told me, looking at Lisa a bit curiously. "But there's some Dillies and Percs over here."

Lisa waited for me in the Carnegie Centre cafeteria while Jeff and I bought a couple dozen pills from a guy on the corner. I wanted to inject them, knowing that would be the fastest way to end my misery. But to do that I'd have to crush them and cook them up. A doable task for, like, five pills. But with this amount, I'd need a soup ladle, a horse needle, and a fat vein. So I dry swallowed them instead. I hoped Lisa was still hanging in there.

"Thanks, Jeff, you saved the day," I said sheepishly.

"No sweat, man," he replied.

On the bus home, I sat with my head in my hands, riding waves of nausea. *Whatever you do*, I told myself, *you gotta hold these pills down*. If I threw up on the bus, I'd just need to score again. Every bump and pothole pushed me right to the edge. Lisa was riding the waves with me, her hand on my knee. She looked worried.

It's way too fucking early for any of this, I thought. *I'm ruining another relationship before it even starts*. But for some reason, I also felt a strange sense of peace.

Back home, I flopped onto the couch. Lisa told me she'd be right back and left my apartment. *She won't be back*, I thought. But I was way too sick to care about that now. I gritted my teeth, praying the pills would kick in soon.

Half an hour later, to my surprise, Lisa buzzed up again. "Hey," she said, setting down grocery bags on the counter. She pulled out some ginger ale, soup and chocolate pudding cups with panda bears on the lids. Next Lisa pulled out a box set of DVDs. She must have stopped at a video store as well.

"Have you seen this?" Lisa asked, holding up a copy of *Peep Show*—a British comedy. "It's great."

I wanted to cry.

For years, whenever I got sick, my biggest priority was being alone. But for some reason I didn't mind that Lisa was here. I lay on the couch, and we laughed along to *Peep Show* until— about half an hour later—my pills finally kicked in. I fell asleep with the TV playing softly in my dreams.

I don't know how long I was out. But when I woke up, I could hardly believe my eyes. My tiny, skittish rescue cat, Stumbles, was purring contentedly in Lisa's lap. Stumbles was frightened of almost everyone. But not Lisa.

She's still here!

"Are you okay?" Lisa asked. The sunlight caught natural red streaks in her hair. I'd never noticed them before. "How are you feeling?"

I listened for any faint trace of judgment in her voice. But I couldn't hear any. She just seemed concerned. I realized that I had never chosen to be with anyone before. Partners had chosen me, or we had ended up together out of happenstance. But I was choosing to be with Lisa, if she'd have me.

"I'm feeling a lot better now," I said. "Thank you."

Over the next few months, Lisa was picking up shifts at a coffee shop in West Vancouver, and I was still working in an office downtown. We met up regularly after work. Sometimes we'd go out to a bar. Other times we'd stay in and watch a movie. I'd only used methadone since the day we scored together. And for some reason, she didn't seem worried that I'd suddenly fall off the wagon.

Lisa and I had been going out for about six months when her roommate moved out. Rents in Vancouver were soaring, and Lisa wouldn't be able to afford her apartment on her own. Should we live together? It seemed a little early, but we were in love. Fuck it. I invited her to move into my place.

Stumbles glued herself to Lisa right away. I was a little hesitant at first, but we spent Christmas at Lisa's parents' house, and her mom made me feel like part of her family. We decorated the tree and gathered around the radio to listen to a reading of Frederick Forsyth's *The Shepherd*. Lisa told me her parents would never judge me, and I could be myself. I was nervous about it, but she was right. They accepted me completely. Lisa's mom called me "one of my chickens."

That same year, Lisa started working on a master's in journalism at UBC, teaching me as she learned. When Lisa had an interview to do, I'd help carry the gear, record sound and edit audio files. She had those skills, but I wanted to be helpful, and this let her focus on the interviewee. Lisa said she liked working with me and suggested that we pitch CBC a radio documentary about albinism.

All over the world, people with albinism faced discrimination. But in several East African countries, there was a gruesome underground market for albino body parts. Rich people bought albino arms and legs, fingers and toes, bones and blood, believing they had magical properties. People with albinism were kidnapped, attacked and murdered. CBC agreed and commissioned our documentary.

Lisa and I got on a plane to St. Louis, where there was an albinism conference. For the first time, I met other people who looked like me. We actually formed a temporary majority there. Lisa had a hard time finding me in a big room full of pale people with white hair.

We interviewed Jane Waithera, an activist with albinism from Kenya. She remembered one time when a man on the street pointed at her. "He said to his friend, 'Look, that's meat—that's banknotes.'" She said East Africans with albinism are often called "zeruzeru," which means "ghost" in Swahili.

We also interviewed Amadou Tidiane Diallo, from Ivory Coast. He told us about being abducted by two men. "I heard one of them saying, 'Oh, this is the meat we were looking for.'" Amadou recounted the story in a quiet voice. "They surrounded me, I fought one of them, one behind knocked me down. I woke up at hospital, didn't know what really happened." Amadou tried to report the incident to the police. "'They were laughing, saying, 'You are a poor albino, you don't need to come and disturb us, we don't have anything to do with people like you. We are here to take charge of people who are normal, you are not a human being.'" At the conference, I heard about how people with albinism were marginalized in North America and Europe, because of disability. There were endless negative TV and movie stereotypes. We were more likely to be poor and unemployed, and I learned that disabled kids experience disproportionate rates of childhood sexual abuse.

I had always found it embarrassing to talk about albinism. But being at the conference with hundreds of people who looked like me made me feel less alone. I was inspired by Jane and Amadou. They were proud survivors, fighting to end violence and discrimination. I needed to leave my shame in St. Louis and join them. I started working with Under the Same Sun, an NGO based in Canada and Tanzania. They hired me to write submissions to the UN about the conditions faced by people with albinism around the world.

The experience brought Lisa and me closer together. And it also brought me closer to my parents, who I interviewed for the documentary. It was the first time we talked openly and at length about their experiences raising a blind kid.

Our documentary "The Imaginary Albino" aired on radio stations across North America. We won a Webster Award and an award at the New York Festivals, where Lisa and I dressed up and attended a gala. The audience gasped when we explained what the documentary was about and then applauded when we accepted the award.

We made documentaries that took us to the Nemaiah Valley in the interior of BC, to London, and to the Giant Mine under Yellowknife. We got to know each other better. We loved travelling together and always found time for fun. On long train rides, I asked her question after question: What were the Balkans like? What were you like as a kid? What drew you to journalism? I wanted to know her whole life story. And Lisa wanted to know mine too. I was a lot less forthcoming than she was, though, deflecting her questions with bad jokes. I told her a little about when I was a kid, but resisted going deeper. "I can't be an open book for you," I finally admitted. "You won't like what you read—I don't even want to read it." Lisa tried her best to understand. "I think I'm broken," I told her, "I think I'm a bad person."

"I don't think that's right," Lisa said. "I see how you take care of the people in your life. You're like being around a horse," she laughed, poking me. "You're big, gentle and calm." I loved the metaphor and whinnied in response. We both laughed, but then Lisa got serious again. She said she'd worked with kids at preschools and summer camps. Hesitantly, she came to her point: "I can see a hurt child in you." I went quiet.

"I think I know someone who can help," Lisa said. She explained that about a year before we started dating, she was on her bike, waiting at a pedestrian crossing on Commercial Drive. An intoxicated driver in a truck blew the light. The truck's side mirror smashed into Lisa's back and broke right off. A couple of inches in the other direction, and Lisa likely would have died. The driver kept going, striking an elderly couple. The woman was left badly injured, bleeding on the road. The man was thrown thirty feet and died.

In the months that followed, Lisa got physiotherapy for her back and hip. But she found herself flashing back to the crash. She was jumpy and hyper-vigilant around traffic, which meant she was jumpy and hyper-vigilant almost everywhere. She was badly traumatized and having serious trouble telling the difference between things that were safe and things that weren't. Recently she had been going to a psychologist for PTSD. "It really helped," she said. "Maybe the therapist can help you too."

I wasn't sure. I told Lisa that I'd been to counselling before and it didn't really help. I told her about the methadone clinic support group. "Nice people," I said, "but the whole thing was kind of useless." But Lisa wasn't saying that I was fucked up or that my brain needed to be fixed. She just wanted me to get the same kind of relief that she had.

"I think it's different if you aren't being forced to go," Lisa said. She explained that her doctor used a technique called eye movement desensitization and reprocessing, or EMDR. "I can't explain it," she said. "It might seem like hippie bullshit, but it sure worked on me." It sounded mysterious, but I said I'd give it a shot.

In Canada's health care system, mental health isn't covered. There were plenty of times when I would never have been able to access this kind of thing. But now that I had a unionized job with extended health coverage, I could swing it. So I booked my first appointment with Dr. Joanne.

"Sit anywhere you like," the doctor told me as I walked into her office. The second-hand, well-worn furniture put me at ease. I chose an armchair and sunk low on its worn-out springs. *What am I doing here?* I wondered, with one eye on the door.

The office was bright, so I kept my sunglasses on. "I've been a junkie for a long time," I told Dr. Joanne, wincing at the sharpness of the word. "It's caused me a lot of problems." I told her that Lisa was the most important person I'd ever met but felt it was just a matter of time before I fucked things up. I didn't want that. I didn't want to wait for dope to come swinging back through my life like a wrecking ball. I didn't want to end up hiding in the bathroom, shooting up. I didn't want to lie about it to Lisa. Now that I had a taste of real happiness, I didn't want to go back to being dopesick, broke and alone.

Dr. Joanne dimmed the lights for me and asked, "Why do you use drugs?" I knew this question was coming, and I had tried to prepare an answer. But instead, I spilled a messy story that wandered through random moments of my life. I told her about being a blind kid in school and about feeling ashamed of my albinism. I told her a little about Victoria, but I couldn't say her name.

At our next session, Dr. Joanne diagnosed me with post-traumatic stress disorder. I was surprised. I thought PTSD was for soldiers, firefighters and residential school survivors. If I had PTSD, then half the planet must have had it too. Dr. Joanne said that PTSD could be treated with EMDR, the therapy Lisa mentioned. "You don't have to relive the events in detail," the doctor said. "You can heal from the bad or traumatic experiences so they become just memories without an emotional charge."

Dr. Joanne handed me a pair of small oval-shaped plastic devices like car key fobs. She told me to hold one in each hand. They were connected by wires to a box that Dr. Joanne held. It looked like a video game controller. She asked me to remember a single image from those bad times. My brain immediately pulled up a picture. I quickly tried to think of something else—*anything* else. But I was stuck on it.

"I'm on some basement stairs . . ." I swallowed. The words were not coming easy. "I don't remember everything. Just fragments." I had the stills. I'd carried them with me since childhood. But the whole video was buried deep. The devices started to buzz, first in my left hand then in my right.

"You don't have to remember everything. Just focus on one image, like one photograph," she said, adjusting the controller. The alternating buzzing sped up.

The image was as clear as the doctor's office.

I'm sitting on the basement stairs. Just stuck there.

The buzzing sped up. Left then right.

There's yellow linoleum on the steps. A pattern of intersecting squares, peeling at one corner.

Buzzing left then right.

A fluorescent light shines down the stairs.

Left.

She's standing at the top of the steps.

Right.

Hands on hips. Red lipstick. Her short platinum hair sticking up.

Buzzing.

Her white coat is open. I look away and trace my finger along the trowel marks in the plaster.

"What are you feeling? And where in your body?" Dr. Joanne asked me.

My throat clamped shut around the words. I felt like I was choking on the memory. Part of me had never moved on. Part of me had seized up and rusted, stuck on the stairs. I couldn't say the name out loud, but the syllables were also too big to swallow.

It all spilled out of me in short, croaking sentences, each one a shocking revelation to me, even though I was saying the words. Victoria saw my loneliness and she weaponized it against me. She was an adult who gave her full attention to a troubled child. She dispensed secret, illicit warmth and acceptance that she knew I craved. She made herself the only source of that warmth, peeling me from my family like the rind of an orange. Then she rationed it, revoked it. She made me feel I was complicit, dirty and alone.

Victoria's naked body made me ashamed of my own. She made me cringe at physical touch. She made me recoil from hugs. For years, I bristled at physical contact from my family. I couldn't hug my grandfather before he died. The distance between me and my parents yawned into adulthood. She made me hate myself.

The buzzing slowed. Dr. Joanne asked, "What do you want to tell that little kid stuck on the stairs?"

It was past and present, all at once—the boy on the stairs and the man in the doctor's office, in superposition. "I want to tell him: 'It's not your fault. You were too young to figure all this out on your own,'" I said.

"You didn't feel safe," the doc said. "Take his hand."

There was no salamander ghost boy anymore. Just a sad, lonely kid in Coke-bottle glasses. A kid that was easy prey. I took the boy's hand, like the doctor said. I led him off the basement stairs. I let go and he walked out into the warm Arctic midnight sun.

The quantum state collapsed. It was just me in the doctor's office, holding some buzzing machines in my hands. There was buzzing in my chest too. My throat opened up. I gulped air. I felt like I was going to throw up. But what came up were sobs. I cried a deluge of long-held-back tears.

My dad worried that I'd have a sad, empty life. So he tried to make me tough. Now I could see that in some ways, I was like him, and like my grandfather. Even in my struggles, I had a little of what was best about them. I thought about Mom. About the silences and gaps between our words, where all the things we should have said to each other had fallen through. All the errors and omissions. Maybe she didn't have the words either. Or maybe I wasn't listening. She spoke in homemade jam, birthday cards and new towels when I moved into a new apartment. Maybe they had their own ghosts. I don't blame them for anything. I realized they never gave up on me.

Leaving the doctor's office, I felt light-headed and dizzy. I stumbled down the corridor, leaning on the walls for support. The tension I'd been holding in my body for decades, in my shoulders, neck and back, was suddenly gone. I wasn't wincing with shame or self-hate. I felt safe, calm and at peace. Lisa was there to pick me up. "Let's go home," she said.

After the appointment I slept for twenty hours straight. Stumbles lay on me, purring like the EMDR machine. I wondered about Stumbles' life before I adopted her from the shelter. Did she have trauma too? I looked at Lisa. This was my family and we would all heal together. Later that week I decided to ask Lisa to marry me.

The Switch

Waiting in the pharmacy, I noticed a poster on the wall. The poster said, "Introducing Methadose™: your new methadone treatment." This wasn't an advertisement: it was an announcement. In a few months—on February 1, 2014—the government would switch all of BC's methadone patients from the generic stuff to a new formulation made by the American pharmaceutical company Mallinckrodt. Over the years I'd heard rumours that American methadone wasn't as good as the Canadian stuff, but I wasn't sure if they were true. "It may look and taste different," the poster explained. "But rest assured, your dose and effect should not change."

As I left the pharmacy with my carries, that weasel word "should" wiggled into my brain. What did they mean? I had used nothing but methadone for over three years and struggled so hard to make methadone work for me. The effect *better* not change. But the poster didn't make it sound like I had an option. I got a bad feeling in my stomach. I was going to be switched—like it or not.

I walked home and paced around. What if the new formulation didn't work as well? What would that mean for my life? For

Jeff's life? I didn't want to just wait around to find out. But what should I do? I asked Lisa what she thought. "Maybe write an article for *Vice* or *Megaphone* or something?" she suggested. "That way you can talk to people who know more about what the new stuff actually is." I liked the idea. I wasn't ready for the world to know I was on methadone, but I figured I wouldn't have to mention that in the article.

That's when I remembered that years ago, at the clinic, someone had handed me a "Patient's Rights" card. It had been in my wallet for ages. I pulled it out and took a closer look. It said that all methadone patients were entitled to respect and dignity and listed some resources I could call if I was getting jerked around. At the top of the card was a picture of a little dragon, the logo for an organization called the British Columbia Association of People on Methadone, or BCAPOM. At the bottom, the card said that BCAPOM met on Wednesdays at the Vancouver Area Network of Drug Users (VANDU) on the 300 block of East Hastings Street. I called the number on the card and asked if I could interview someone from the group. The person who answered told me, "You need to talk to Laura Shaver."

A few days later, Lisa and I walked down to VANDU in rare November sunshine. As we opened the door to the storefront, a terrible scraping sound assaulted my ears. Someone was setting out chairs into rows for a meeting, dragging the metal legs across the floor. I looked around. There were a couple of well-worn couches—a guy was taking a nap on one. A woman behind the front counter handed new rigs and pipes to a couple. The walls were covered with a riot of images: posters for demonstrations, bad drug alerts and a "No dealing on the premises" sign. A flower-emblazoned banner hung from the ceiling. It read, "In memory of our members who lost their lives to the drug war." There were dozens of photos of smiling faces on the walls. I realized that they were memorials, tributes to drug user activists who'd died. I could tell that this was a revolutionary space: a place for fighting back.

The woman behind the counter told me I'd find Laura upstairs in her office. I poked my head into a room, unsure if I was in the right place. "Are you Laura?" I asked.

"You betcha!" said a woman with strawberry-blonde hair and sunglasses pushed back on her head. Laura came around a desk overflowing with notebooks and policy manuals. Her office was a bit of a squirrel's nest, but I got the impression Laura could put her hands on whatever file she wanted in seconds.

"I'm on methadone," I told Laura as Lisa plugged in a mic and got levels on her recorder. My throat was tight and my voice sounded a bit choked. I was nervous, but Laura seemed relaxed. She apologized for having to eat between meetings. "You obviously know a lot more about the changes coming to the methadone program," I said.

"The thing that's driving me nuts is we have no choice," Laura said, explaining that she'd been meeting with the officials running the methadone program. Laura said she'd told them, "You can't just spring it on us," but they'd politely brushed her off.

"Do we know what this new stuff actually is?" I asked. Laura nodded. Methadose was a widely prescribed formulation of methadone in the US, she explained. Generic Canadian methadone was a kind of powder that pharmacists mixed into a

Tang-flavoured juice. The new Methadose was a pre-mixed cherry-flavoured syrup. Laura said she thought the main benefit of the new stuff—from the government's perspective—was that it would be harder for crooked pharmacists to dilute and sell out the back door.

"One of the biggest things about the new methadone is that it's ten times stronger," Laura told me. "Which means if you're on 150 millilitres of methadone, say, then when you take Methadose, you will only take 15 millilitres."

"Do you think it's going to lead to more overdoses and deaths?" I asked.

"Oh yes. I'm sure of it," Laura replied. Plenty of people buy methadone illegally on the street. If someone just took the amount they were used to, they'd end up with ten times the effect and could easily overdose.

"What can we do about it?" I asked. Laura told me that she and some others at BCAPOM had offered to test the new stuff on themselves. Even though they didn't want to be switched, they were willing to try it early if the government was determined to switch *everyone*. There were around fifteen thousand methadone patients in the province, and Laura cared more about their safety than her own health. But she said the government had turned her down.

Who is this person? I thought. Laura appeared to embody two extremes. On the one hand, she seemed like some kind of policy insider. She was squeezing this interview into a busy schedule of meetings and phone calls. She explained that a big part of her role was to help other drug users navigate the Byzantine methadone system. She was comfortable talking about the chemical composition of methadone, the social life of drug users and the frustrating mechanics of federal and provincial policy making.

On the other hand, Laura seemed like a total badass. She had been through the shit and she was proud to have survived. "See this?" Laura asked, pointing to a scar on her forehead. She explained she got it from a stint in hospital when she was deeply dopesick. She saw a nurse passing by with a cart full of pills. Hoping for some relief, Laura said she made a dive for the pills, but ended up crashing headfirst into the cart instead. Laura laughed as she told the story—there was a sheer lack of shame in her voice. I couldn't help but laugh too. We had a lot in common—as methadone patients and activists. *I like her,* I thought.

Laura explained she'd grown up Mormon in Kelowna. She rode horses as a kid and played basketball in high school. She got into dope around that time and was prescribed methadone at nineteen. "I was told I was the youngest person in British Columbia to ever be on the program," she said, her voice hinting at something that almost seemed like pride to me. Methadone was hard work, Laura said. But after years she was finally able to stop using heroin. She had a child who'd been taken from her, she added. She wanted to regain custody one day. And she knew she'd never get there without success on the methadone program.

I thought about how different Laura's story was from all those redemption yarns I'd heard at twelve-step meetings. She wasn't a sinner who'd been saved. There was no flash of insight from her Higher Power and she wasn't trying to get off methadone. She wasn't driven by a constant desire to kick, like I had been. This wasn't giving up, this was self-acceptance.

She explained that the main benefit of methadone was that it was legal and subsidized. To Laura, heroin was dangerous *because* it was illegal and expensive. Unlike regulated drugs such as methadone, you could never be sure how potent the heroin you bought off the street actually was. The drug war drove up heroin's price as well—enriching organized crime and impoverishing drug users. People had to resort to risky and dangerous schemes to support their habits.

I recognized the truth in Laura's story and felt its relevance to my own life. I was still planning to keep the fact that I was on methadone a secret from whoever wound up reading or hearing this interview. But part of me yearned to let the secret go. I wanted to learn how to speak with the same kind of confidence that Laura had. I wanted to stop hating myself. We'd only been talking for about half an hour, and Laura already had me questioning the story I'd been telling myself for years about my own drug.

"You should come to a BCAPOM meeting," Laura said. She handed me a poster she'd made warning about the upcoming methadone switch. Laura explained that BCAPOM members had been hanging them up around East Vancouver, on pharmacy bulletin boards and lampposts. If I was worried about people getting switched, then I should join the struggle.

"I'll be there," I told her. I still didn't know how to summon the kind of bravery that Laura had. BCAPOM was a very public group. They did interviews with the media and put on demonstrations. And all their members were methadone users. I figured if I joined it would just be a matter of time before someone rec-ognized me and realized that I was on methadone too. *That's not as important as warning people about the switch*, I told myself. The next week, I attended my first BCAPOM meeting. I was finally joining the fight.

I took a seat near the back on one of the noisy, floor-scraping chairs. A guy with long hair and a bowler hat was working his way through the rows, taking names for a list. About thirty people were there, mostly men. Many gave street names like "Superman" and "Drop-D." When he asked me, I didn't give a pseudonym. I said Garth. He wrote it down and introduced himself as Al Fowler. We chatted for a few min-utes. Al was on the BCAPOM board of directors and had been an activist for several years. He lived a few blocks from me with his wife, Nicole, and his cat, Baby Girl. He told me that Nicole liked to put the cat in fancy little doll dresses.

"What does the cat think of that?" I asked.

"She puts up with it," Al laughed.

Right at two o'clock, Al stood and started a roll call of the attendees and then sat behind a desk with Laura and three others, including Chereece Keewatin, Laura's best friend and the group's vice-president. Chereece read the group's mission statement: "To support, protect and defend methadone patients' rights to live free from obstacles caused by addiction and prejudice." Then Laura addressed the group. "For those of you who are new, or may have missed this information, we're talk-ing about Methadose again today." Hands shot up. People asked what it was, when the switch was coming and how we could stop it.

I continued to attend the Wednesday meetings and met others from the wider VANDU community. In the past, I thought it might not be possible for drug users to get organized. But now it was happening all around me. VANDU was a place where we could build the kind of community we needed to stay safe. It was a place where we could find real meaning— where we could be part of something bigger than ourselves. Most of the VANDU old-timers I met credited this kind of connection with saving their lives.

One day I told Hugh Lampkin, a VANDU board member, that I was starting to feel the same way. That this place was giving me an important new kind of meaning. He said that most members had a story like mine. "VANDU is a place of redemption," he told me earnestly. "No matter who you were before, this is where you become who you were supposed to be." He added, "As we make the world new, we make ourselves new too."

I kicked myself for having taken so long to get here.

On the first of February, the switch began. As the prescriptions of fifteen thousand methadone patients gradually ran out, their doctors wrote new ones for Methadose. My script was due to run out at the end of the month, so I was anxious to hear from people who'd already tried the new stuff. I wanted to know how it was going.

I asked Laura, who'd just made the switch. She had initially been worried that concentrated Methadose might be too strong. But now she said, "It doesn't have legs." Laura explained that Methadose started out okay for her, but it petered out long before it was time for her next dose. "I woke up feeling like my legs were moving, I couldn't sleep, and I felt twitches," Laura said. She lay in bed panicking about what was going to happen next. "I'm going to be doing heroin," she said to me, starting to cry. "That means I am going to be robbing jewellery stores. That means I am going to be in jail." I could feel Laura's usual self-assuredness melt away, and I realized Laura wasn't immune to the kind of shame I still felt deep down. She'd built herself up with the right kind of medicine, but now the government was taking that away. Laura knew it wouldn't be long before her life unravelled.

And it wasn't just Laura who'd noticed. I met Jeff down the street at the Ovaltine Cafe. We sat in our regular booth and ordered bacon and eggs. Jeff was looking more haggard than normal. I asked him if he'd been switched yet. He nodded. "The new juice is garbage," he said. Like Laura, Jeff said he was getting severe withdrawal symptoms before it was time for his next dose. Jeff estimated that Methadose only lasted him about sixteen hours. "It comes on hard and fast, then dies quick," he explained. As Jeff described his first night on Methadose, I felt prickles of fear in my scalp. He said he was sick and sweating at three a.m., "the spider crawling up and down my spine." Jeff told me he saw a grim future flash in front of him. "I'll be back to robbing banks," he said, picking at his eggs.

Fuck, I thought. How many people was this happening to?

Jeff came with me to the next BCAPOM meeting. Like me, he wanted to reverse the switch. Looking around, I noticed how sick many seemed. People were clamouring over each other and Chereece called on us to quiet down. Then, one by one, BCAPOM members shared their nearly identical stories.

"I told my doc the new stuff ain't holding me," one user said. "But he just wouldn't believe me."

"Has anyone else tried talking to their doctor about this?" Laura asked. Several hands went up. "And how'd that go?" People had been told different things: "It will just take a while to adjust to." Or, "That's weird, it should be chemically identical to the old stuff." But the result was the same in every case: people were kept on Methadose, even though it wasn't working for them. I wasn't surprised. Doctors don't believe drug users almost as a rule.

"And how are you doing now?" Laura asked. The stories started to get grimmer: people were using heroin again, they were doing sex work again, they were stealing stuff, their families and friends were mad at them. I knew it wouldn't be long before my prescription was up as well. I had no idea what I'd do. I was terrified that my worst-case scenario was coming true: dopesickness was coming for me. If I was too sick to show up for work, I'd lose my job. Then I'd lose my housing. I didn't want to put Lisa through this and risk losing her too. I started to feel that it was naive to have ever trusted the stability I'd found on methadone. It could be taken away from me in an instant.

My script ran out in late February. I had an appointment with Dr. M and told her how worried I was that the new stuff wouldn't work for me. I asked her if she'd noticed anything weird happening to her patients who'd switched to Methadose. "Yes," she said. Many had become "less stable" since the switch. She didn't seem to be a fan of the new medication and told me she had no idea why this change was being made.

"Am I right that you have to travel frequently for work?" Dr. M said.

"Yes I do," I answered. I had to travel to several remote locations in BC that winter, and only small amounts of liquids were permitted in airplane carry-on baggage. Nothing over one hundred millilitres. And my carries were much more than that.

"Methadone tablets are recommended for carry-on luggage," she explained. "Can you please give the clinic copies of your boarding passes or other documentation?"

"No problem," I said. I photocopied plane tickets and itineraries. Since Methadose was not available in tablets, Dr. M prescribed me Metadol pills instead. I tried them, and they felt just like the old methadone. At BCAPOM, I suggested that others ask their doctors, but nobody seemed to have any success.

That rainy winter, I could almost feel dopesickness rippling across the province. Each week, there were fewer and fewer members at BCAPOM's Wednesday meetings. Even some of the elected board were MIA. They were dopesick and out grinding for money to get well. They didn't have time to be sitting in a meeting. Laura asked me to join the BCAPOM board of directors and help organize a campaign to get the old methadone back. I joined Chereece, Laura and Al for a series of meetings with the constellation of bureaucrats responsible for the methadone system.

Soon I'd been to a dozen of these meetings. Everyone was always dressed West Coast business casual. They showed us

PowerPoints in various boardrooms. We got soft-spoken empathy and crocodile tears, but never any action.

There was also plenty of finger-pointing and buck-passing in these meetings. The bureaucrats kept making it seem like *nobody* had been in charge of the switch and nobody had the power to reverse it. Each department, ministry and agency had its own rules and budgets, they explained. I started to realize that this kind of diffusion of responsibility was the government's phantom power—a way to shield them from their actions. And the only way to fight it was to dive into the minutiae. I was becoming a policy analyst here too.

At BCAPOM meetings, members suggested that maybe the government would actually listen if we had someone else on our side. A lawyer maybe. Or better yet a scientist. Someone who could prove that this was *actually* happening. That it wasn't all in our heads. "I think I know someone," Laura said. At the next BCAPOM meeting Laura introduced us to Dr. Ryan McNeil. Ryan was an assistant professor at the UBC Faculty of Medicine and he ran the qualitative unit at the BC Centre on Substance Use. He was the real deal. But in a ball cap, beard and hoodie, Ryan didn't look like a suit. For the past several years, he'd worked with VANDU to publish papers on needle exchanges, supervised injection, peer-run programs, HIV and police misconduct. His research topics were informed by what was important to VANDU. This was more than a career for Ryan. He seemed to really care about drug users.

When we explained what was happening, Ryan told us that this was an important moment to gather data, as the switch was still in its first few months. Ryan designed a study and Chereece was named as a co-author on the paper, which was published in the journal *Social Science & Medicine*. I opened the paper, the master's degree part of me, the activist part and the dopefiend part all reading together: "The introduction of Methadose precipitated increased withdrawal symptoms [and] . . . re-initiation of injection drug use and participation in high-risk income-generating strategies."

When Ryan explained the results of the study to a BCAPOM meeting, I could feel the room vibrate with a sense of vindication. The group had experienced the switch themselves, up close. But for most of us, seeing it written down in black and white made it feel more real. The one exception was Jeff. "I fuckin' told ya," he said, "no need to do a study."

I sent the BC Ministry of Health Ryan's study. They dismissed it due to its small sample size. Professor Alissa Greer from Simon Fraser University published a paper surveying 405 methadone patients. Half of the respondents reported using multiple substances after the switch to deal with withdrawal symptoms.

I sent the government Greer's study too, and they said the sample size was still too small. Why was it on us to prove this anyway? There was something else going on here. This wasn't about quibbles over methodology. This was dismissing us, even when we had evidence. By the time M. Eugenia Socías published another paper showing "immediate increases in illicit heroin injection" after the switch, I knew it wouldn't matter. We asked Ryan McNeil to start attending government meetings with us to summarize the research. But still nobody believed us. "It's all in your head," they said.

History Repeating

plugged my ears as two ambulances wailed down Hastings Street. A scratchy haze hung over the city from the climate-change-fuelled mega-wildfires that had become a regular part of summer. The blood-red sun gave the city an apocalyptic feel. My sleeveless T-shirt stuck to my back. The single-room occupancy hotels were too hot to stay in, so everyone sat out on the street. Wu-Tang played from a boom box somewhere.

Was I hearing more sirens lately? Inside VANDU, I poured myself a cup of coffee from the shiny metal urn near the front desk. On the rare times when someone made coffee, it always had sugar and powdered whitener added in. I usually took it black, but I liked the weird chemical coffee whitener. The woman sitting behind the desk asked if I knew two guys who hung around Oppenheimer Park. "I don't think so," I said. "They both died recently," she responded, and pointed to a bad dope alert posted on the wall. It warned of a brown powder which was sold as heroin but tested positive for fentanyl. "Be careful," she said.

I flashed back to the 1990s. I remembered the overdoses, funerals, sirens, newspaper headlines. I felt light-headed. This couldn't be happening again—it couldn't. Does everything really come back around? I wondered what had happened to those two guys. They'd gone to take their normal shot and . . . what? Just fell on the ground.

I'd used fentanyl before, with Jeff. I remember when I first tried it how excited I felt to get my hands on something *stronger* than heroin. But I didn't really like it. For whatever reason, fentanyl didn't give me the feeling I was after. It wasn't a warm blanket. Maybe the risk had less to do with the actual drug and more to do with the potency. It was the not knowing that killed you.

I knew that there were advantages to fentanyl from the dealers' perspective. Heroin had to be smuggled across the world from poppy fields in Mexico, Colombia or Afghanistan. But you could make fentanyl in a lab in Vancouver or buy it from overseas on the dark web. And because fentanyl was so potent, you could make the same amount of money by moving way less weight. It was an old pattern. When cops cracked down, dealers had to find something smaller and more powerful. That's how we got from opium to heroin and then China White. "The harder the enforcement, the harder the drugs," as the Iron Law of Prohibition said. Fent was going to be big. It was simple economics.

At the next BCAPOM meeting, other drug user activists echoed my concerns. We had a tradition of ending each meeting with a moment of silence. Everyone would whisper the names of people they'd lost to the drug war. It seemed like we all had more names to say than normal. And more of those names were *recent* deaths. In the year of the switch, overdose deaths started creeping back up to what they were during the last crisis, in the 1990s. We held services at VANDU and made regular trips to Glenhaven Memorial Chapel. "Methadose and fentanyl are a one-two punch taking us out," Laura said.

Being an activist at VANDU felt like being plugged into a grim Distant Early Warning system. Laura knew she was in danger. Chereece knew she was in danger. Jeff was in danger, though he was loath to admit it. And—if I was being honest with myself—I knew I was in danger too. I had gone four years without using anything other than methadone. But there were times when that wasn't easy. I knew there was always the possibility I would slip up and chip. And if that happened, it would be like playing Russian roulette. Again. But I was especially worried about all my friends who *weren't* part of the drug user movement. All the punks I'd come up with had no idea what was coming.

Jeff was living back in the neighbourhood, at the Washington Hotel. I sat on his bed while he paced his ten-by-ten-foot room. "How's it going?" I asked.

"Shitty," he said, handing me a small slip of paper that had clearly been crumpled up and then smoothed out again. I squinted down at rows of tiny doctor handwriting. Jeff realized that I couldn't read it and cut to the chase.

"I'm getting cut off," he explained. Jeff's doctor was tapering his slow-release oral morphine pills right down to nothing. In the wake of the Methadose switch, Jeff's pain pills had managed to keep him safe from the illicit supply. But now he was losing the morphine as well.

"What are you gonna do?" I asked.

"Be sick as fuck," Jeff said. "I'll have to go back to work. With garbage juice and no pills, what the fuck else can I do? I'll need dope." Jeff was going back to subsistence dope dealing to support his habit.

"It's not just happening to me," Jeff added. "She's cutting everyone in the clinic off their pain pills." I knew the clinic Jeff was talking about. Many BCAPOM members were patients there.

I nodded grimly. I'd followed the first wave of news stories. A full-blown panic was sweeping the US over "hillbilly heroin," the media's name for Oxycodone. These stories blamed doctors for overprescribing pain medications. In Canada and the US, officials were rolling out new patient and physician surveillance tools to limit access to pills. Doctors were cutting off their patients, who then went to score dope off the streets instead—and that's when the bodies really started piling up.

At the next meeting, I asked Laura if BCAPOM could write a letter to the doctor on behalf of the members who were cut off. Laura emailed the doctor that evening: "Hi Doctor, How are you doing? It has been brought to our attention that people are being taken off their pain medications which of course turns people's lives into a twist. Some people cannot handle it. Is there a certain reason for this?"

The next week, Laura read out the doctor's response. The doctor was worried about side effects of ongoing morphine prescribing. She wrote, "I want to be really supportive for people to find non-medication ways to lessen their pain such as swimming, exercise, or mindfulness." Laura stopped reading. Chereece scoffed, repeating, "Swimming?"

———

In 2015, more people died from fatal overdoses in BC than in any single year during the crisis in the 1990s. By 2016, fentanyl had started to overtake heroin on the streets. It was street fentanyl—not prescription pills—that was causing the huge increase in deaths.

It seemed hard to believe. This city, where once I could score high-quality dope day or night, had almost completely run out of heroin. I hoped that once everyone gained a tolerance for fent, the deaths would stop. But illicit fentanyl proved to be far more volatile than heroin. Just when you thought you'd gotten used to the stuff, you'd encounter a poorly mixed batch and your number was up.

Jeff had found peace with the old methadone and slow-release oral morphine and had even stopped using down. But all that was history now, and Jeff had a big habit to support. In the past, he'd sold dope or worked as a Six Man—a lookout for someone selling drugs on the street. Now Jeff was supplied by a dealer who he paid back at the end of each day. He was careful not to get in debt, but he could never get ahead either. Still, Jeff had a code: he didn't sling contaminated dope, and used drug checking services to confirm the quality of the product.

No matter how bad the dope got, people were going to use anyway. I did. Activists pleaded with the government to offer a safe alternative to toxic street drugs. Expand the prescription heroin program, we demanded. Enable access to regulated drugs with a known, predictable potency. Return to the old methadone. Reinstate pain pill prescriptions. But time and time again, the government refused. Nobody was coming to save us. We realized that we'd have to save ourselves.

The lineup at Insite, Canada's first legal supervised injection site, was always long. So Ann Livingston and former Park Board commissioner Sarah Blyth put up a tent in an alley. Inside, people could shoot up, and Ann and Sarah had naloxone and the training to reverse any overdoses. Stephen Harper's Conservative government had practically outlawed this kind of life-saving effort, so they did it illegally, just like Ann had done twenty years earlier. But this time—amidst the shocking amount of death—the government didn't crack down on the operation. Eventually, the Vancouver Coastal Health Authority permitted VANDU to open a small room in the back of the storefront. Our members supervised each other with naloxone and oxygen tanks at the ready. Across the Downtown Eastside, drug users were resuscitating each other.

It was a cold winter for this city. VANDU activists patrolled snowy alleys, looking for anyone slumped over. Too often, people would shoot dope alone behind the Washington Hotel. And all too often, bodies were found in the slush.

I was lying in bed on the morning of April 14, 2016, half awake, half asleep, listening to the radio. I needed to get up, take my methadone and go to work. The hourly news came on. BC's provincial health officer, Perry Kendall, had just declared a public health emergency due to rapidly increasing overdose deaths. I sat bolt upright, putting my feet over the side of the bed. The cat sat up too, her ears pointing at me like antennae.

"What's going on?" Lisa asked sleepily.

"It's official," I said. "Again." I couldn't believe it. This was going to be my second formally declared drug war mass death event. Memories of the 1990s surged up in me like bile.

Before long, it was the biggest news story in the country. The chief coroner started reporting death statistics every month. Nearly a thousand died that year. The next year, 1,500 died. Old-school heroin veterans with decades-long habits were dropping like flies. The best people in our movement were disappearing, with barely enough time to memorialize their lives before the next death: Tracey Morrison was a VANDU leader and the neighbourhood's "Bannock Lady," Lori Preston was a BCAPOM board member who always made a nice Christmas dinner for her friends, and Charlie Boyle was BCAPOM's treasurer. Over a couple years, so many people had died that VANDU was losing its ability to function. "Who can take notes well around here now?" "Who's good with computers?" "Who can talk to the media?" Everyone scrambled to learn the skills that had died with our friends and comrades.

In 2017, the old, right-leaning BC Liberal government was thrown out, and I was glad to see them go. Newly elected premier John Horgan and his New Democratic Party government promised action on the overdose crisis. They created a new Ministry of Mental Health and Addictions. But Dean Wilson, an early VANDU leader, cautioned me to not hold my breath. "The NDP has never done fuck all for drug users," he said, recalling inaction the last time they'd been in power, almost twenty years earlier.

I knew Dean had a point, but I hoped the new government might do something about our methadone situation. I emailed a request to meet with the new addiction minister, Judy Darcy. Six months later, Darcy was finally ready to talk, and I went to her Vancouver office with Laura and Chereece. We explained how Methadose and fentanyl were tearing our lives apart. Laura told the minister about what had happened to her since the switch. How the stability she had on methadone was ripped away from her. How she was using down now and worried about overdosing. Chereece started to cry. She told Darcy about how hard she'd fought to get off heroin and how the switch had stolen that from her. I stared at Darcy intently. She seemed like a normal, compassionate human being. *How can anyone hear this stuff and not be moved to act?* I wondered.

When it was my turn to talk, I told Darcy that the switch was driving a lot of the overdose deaths. We needed to give people their old methadone back as soon as possible. But—I added—that wouldn't be enough. People were now wired to illicit fentanyl, and I knew that for many, methadone wasn't going to be strong enough to address that kind of habit. We needed to give people on-demand access to diacetylmorphine (heroin) as well. Even to pharmaceutical fentanyl. Echoing a new consensus amongst drug user activists across the country, I told Darcy that access to these kinds of pharmaceutical drugs would get us out of the crisis. "You have to act now," I said. "The window to save lives is closing fast."

We knew that the ministry barely had a budget of its own and likely couldn't act unilaterally. But we told the minister that we hoped she could take our concerns to Adrian Dix,

BC's minister of health. Or better yet, to Premier John Horgan. Minister Darcy listened and nodded. She seemed genuinely moved by our stories and said that we should meet again. But our follow-up meetings were with her junior staff, not with officials in a position to make any kind of real policy changes.

For three years, VANDU and BCAPOM did everything we could think of to reduce the number of deaths. We saved lives ourselves, rescuing people we found passed out on the street. We leafleted clinics. We held demonstrations. We occupied the atrium of the building where Health Canada's offices were located. We gave interviews to the media. We lobbied the government. In the massive scope of the drug war, amidst the rising tide of deaths, we sought the smallest unit of change imaginable: access to a formulation of methadone that had been available for decades. But we were stonewalled at every turn.

In the chaos of the overdose crisis, I'd barely noticed how drug user activism was taking over my life. I was spending as much time organizing as I spent at my day job. A lot of my friends were in the movement now. These relationships were vital to me, but they could also be brutal. As Laura and I grew closer, I watched her struggle to hang on to the things she'd worked so hard to build: her political fire, her stability, her relationship, her happiness and her dream of reconciliation with her daughter. In the years following the switch, Laura would overdose nine times. On one occasion, I found her slumped in a chair in her office. She had no colour and her face was slack. I thought she was dead. She came around, but it was a close call.

Laura's life was rocked by Methadose and by fentanyl, yet she continued to fight for all of us. I was even more in awe of her now than when we first met. And her radical self-acceptance was rubbing off on me. Now when I told people I was on methadone, I said it like her. With pride in my voice. I was learning how to stoke that same kind of fire in myself.

Transmission

t had been about a year since we'd started holding meetings for the *Crackdown* podcast project, and I was starting to worry: were we ever going to actually make a radio show? Or were we just going to keep sitting around talking about it? Maybe we hired the wrong people. Maybe this was a bad plan all along. How did we get here?

The idea came from Ryan McNeil originally. Like me, Ryan was fed up with the way the mainstream media was covering the overdose crisis. Too often, they wrote about the crisis like a force of nature, rarely pausing to consider the real causes and possible solutions—other than policing. Conservative columnists called us scumbags, zombies and junkies. If reporters were feeling generous, they called us addicts, but that still felt like a slap in the face. Often, we were included in articles as a cautionary tale, or a note of pathos, not as experts who might actually have some answers. A few journalists were doing right by us, but for the most part, we were blamed or pitied, but never given any agency.

Ryan and I were both frustrated that no one was covering the Methadose story, so there was little pressure on the BC government to give us the old methadone back. "I think maybe we could do a better job if we just did this ourselves," Ryan said. "We could do a podcast."

I'd also wondered if podcasting could be more effective at getting the drug user movement's message out there than the kind of short print stories I was writing. Maybe we could say more this way. Maybe there wouldn't be so many gatekeepers.

I told Ryan that if we were going to do this, I was happy to be the show's host and share a little of my life. But I didn't want the show to just be about me and didn't want to speak on behalf of all drug users. So Ryan and I set to work at forming an editorial board of drug user activists from various parts of the movement and with a wide range of experiences. Some names came right away. Of course Jeff had to be there. He knew this world better than anyone. And Laura, Chereece and Al should all be on the board too. I asked Dean Wilson, the first person ever to use at Insite and someone I considered to be an elder statesman of the movement. We asked Shelda Kastor to join. Shelda was on the board of the Western Aboriginal Harm Reduction Society. We asked Samona Marsh, who had been president of VANDU. We also approached Dave Murray, a walking encyclopedia of prescribed heroin programs around the world, and we asked Greg Fresz. Both were part of the lucky hundred or so who were participants in a prescribed heroin study and continued to get it at the Crosstown Clinic. With this group, we'd be able to do movement journalism. We'd support the drive for change instead of just reporting on events from a neutral distance.

Our first meeting truly started at square one. "What's a podcast?" someone asked. Half our editorial board didn't have internet access. "It's like radio but on the computer," I explained. "We can't let it suck," someone else said, followed by a clamour of agreement. People always treated drug users like we were kids. We knew that if we made something below average, we'd be given a patronizing pat on the head just for trying. And no one wanted that. "Let's make this thing actually good." We tossed around names, including some really bad ones, like "Talking Smack" and "Heroin Radio," but then Taylor Fleming, a coordinator working with Ryan, suggested "Crackdown." We knew right away it was the perfect name.

Lisa and I had a frank conversation about the show later that night. Did we have time to do this by ourselves? The vision for the show was steadily growing, from a handful of interviews to an audio documentary series. Lisa had made short radio reports in the Balkans and together we'd made one-hour documentaries, but never an ongoing series. We were both already working full-time jobs. We needed to find some hired guns.

I thought back to some podcasters I'd met at the Webster Journalism Awards. They'd made a documentary about the clinic where Dave and Greg received prescribed heroin. My first meeting with Sam Fenn and Alex Kim was held in a boardroom Ryan had booked. Sam was a redhead in his early thirties, with a loud voice. Alex—who was still in his twenties—was quieter. The guys came in wearing button-up shirts and flaunting a pitch deck. They had production chops, but I didn't want to hire slick producers. I wanted comrades. We took a chance on them anyway.

Months later, when we finally released *Crackdown*'s first episode, I wondered if this had all been a mistake. We had spent ages talking about a million little details—the show's logo, the format, the "contract with the listener." Sam seemed genuinely passionate about the show, but I knew we were one of about four clients he was working with at the time. *Crackdown*'s first episode was an introduction to the podcast—"the drug war, covered by drug users as war correspondents." We published it on the web, and waited to see what would happen.

The month *Crackdown* launched, it seemed like the media was more focused on the drug war than I could ever remember. The overdose crisis was national headline news. We sent out press releases to promote our new show, and to my surprise, the requests for interviews came pouring in. The morning our first episode went live, I was interviewed for CBC Radio's national morning show, *The Current*.

Everything started to click on the show's second episode. Our editorial board was unanimous: We needed to do a story about the methadone switch. Over the next few days, Alex and Sam peppered me with questions: What is methadone actually supposed to *do*? What does dopesickness actually feel like? What's heroin like compared to methadone? What is fentanyl like? Why are so many people dying?

As the story became clearer to Sam and Alex, I could tell they were actually moved. "Jesus," Sam said. "I didn't know any of this." Alex had a habit of letting Sam do the talking, but I could tell by his face that something had changed for him as well. The podcaster guys were furious about what had happened to us and determined to do whatever it took to get other people to care.

Sam and Alex asked me to think of someone I knew who wasn't affiliated with BCAPOM. Someone who couldn't have seen the switch coming. I said that my friend Ray was like that.

"What was his life like before Methadose?" the guys asked.

"Pretty good," I responded. I knew Ray had a construction job and played guitar in a local punk band. I also knew that Ray's life had been destroyed by the switch.

A few days later, I interviewed Ray. Sitting on a park bench, he told me about how he'd become a journeyman carpenter thanks to the stability of methadone. He remembered hating the taste of Methadose the first time he tried it. But, when he started getting dopesick, he didn't think to blame the new stuff. "This might be psychological," he said. Or maybe it had something to do with his bad liver. Either way, after a few days of excruciating withdrawal, Ray found a number for a dealer he hadn't used in years. All of his work to rebuild his life around methadone started to crumble without him ever understanding what had happened. At the end of the interview, Ray picked up a battered old guitar and sang "Moonshiner," a folk song about the experience of addiction. As snow fell around us, his voice was on the verge of cracking and his cold hands struggled to hold the chords.

I've played plenty of gigs where only the people in the other bands turn up, and I figured *Crackdown* would probably be the same. I imagined a few dozen listeners. But we shot right to the top of the Canada iTunes charts. *Canadaland* would describe us as "the best new podcast in Canada." Journalists and other podcasters called for interviews. The *Vancouver Sun* and *Megaphone* ran features. We were covered by the *Columbia Journalism Review* and J-Source. We were flooded with social media posts and messages.

It turned out that plenty of drug users listened to our show. People told me they felt seen, they felt less alone, and they wished they had a VANDU in their town. "*Crackdown* is such an incredible podcast," one listener wrote as a review. "It brings me so much joy and has helped heal my misconceptions, stigmas, and general knowledge of drugs and how they work."

But the most important reaction came from VANDU, from the people who the show was about. We held a listening party and people sat in rapt attention, listening closely to every word. I'd never seen the place so focused. There was laughter and applause. When we asked for feedback, someone said, "We're pretty hilarious people, so keep it funny."

Looking back, it's amazing how much of the *Crackdown* formula was already in place while we worked on the show's second episode. This was movement journalism—driven by drug user activists. We were telling stories that only people in the life knew about. It was narrative. It had a first-person perspective: I wrote and interviewed *as a drug user*, relating the stories back to my own experience. *Crackdown* was also serious investigative journalism. We held powerful people accountable for what was happening to us.

Crackdown also had a unique sound. We left in as many human moments as possible. And we gradually learned to write in a house style—with Sam, Alex, Lisa and me jumping over each other to make each line as direct, forceful and honest as possible. Sam and I recorded feedback-drenched guitars to score our episodes. And, later, a local musician named James Ash filled out our sound with beautiful synth textures.

Each person on the production team brought their own skills. Lisa had journalism, Sam had story structure, and Alex had sound design. Eventually, journalist Alex de Boer joined our ranks, bringing a deep commitment to local politics and history. I brought a lifetime of surviving prohibition.

I started to feel comfortable with my role. All the different parts of me had been at war. But now the punk rocker, musician, organizer, policy wonk and dopefiend sides of me were all working together. Behind the mic, I was starting to become my true self.

We wanted listeners to trust what we said, and our enemies would sink us if we slipped up. We had to get everything correct. That started with street knowledge, but we fact-checked our scripts rigorously and made sure our words were backed up by academic research. That was Ryan McNeil's area of expertise. Not only was he one of the show's co-founders, he was our science director as well, making sure we had the relevant studies and helping us interpret them. He introduced us to his colleagues, and many of them came on board. Thomas Kerr, Jade Boyd and Danya Fast are world-leading experts in drug policy research with a tower of peer-reviewed papers under their names.

I dove into the research, but now I asked my questions to Ryan on the mic, instead of by text. One day over beers, Ryan asked if I'd ever thought about going back to school. I said I was interested, and he supported my application to UBC's Interdisciplinary Studies Graduate Program. I was going to be a student again.

Lisa made arrangements with the health authority so that *Crackdown* could become its own satellite harm reduction site.

We started giving out naloxone kits, and Lisa and I began training everyone who had anything to do with *Crackdown* on how to reverse overdoses. Then we started training students at her college. Lisa's students reported using their new skills to save lives. Soon other schools and workplaces requested we come in. Eventually, we had trained hundreds of people. *Crackdown* was becoming more than a podcast; it was becoming a community.

Everything was coming together, and I was starting to feel good. But then, on February 21, 2019, I got the news. I was at the offices of the BC Centre on Substance Use. Dr. Evan Wood pulled me aside, guiding me to a private spot. When we were alone, Evan said, "I'm sorry to tell you this, Garth. Chereece is gone. It happened last night."

It felt like a cinder block had been hurled at my stomach. The air left me and I doubled over, just like I did when I first got the wind knocked out of me by another kid when I was eight.

"Fuck," I gasped.

"It's okay. Take your time."

"How'd it happen?"

Evan shrugged. He meant, "You know how. Overdose."

I called Laura as soon as I could. When she answered the phone, she sounded like a wounded animal. We met at the Main Street SkyTrain station and hugged. Laura began crying so hard that she struggled to breathe. I wrapped my army parka around her, and slowly her breathing returned to normal. We stood like that for forty-five minutes.

"I have no doubt the switch is what killed her," Laura said. I asked if we should hit pause on the Methadose episode.

"Hell no," she said. "This story is about Chereece. It's about all of us. And it needs to be told. The crisis doesn't stop, and neither do we."

We dedicated our second episode to Chereece Keewatin and vowed to keep fighting to get justice for her death.

I was a little surprised to see Laura at the next BCAPOM meeting. We were all shell-shocked; Chereece had been a fixture around VANDU for years. Now her chair next to Laura sat empty.

Things had changed in the five years since the switch in February 2014. They had been hard years for everyone. We still had to get the old methadone back, but that wasn't going to be enough anymore. The old formulation made a pretty good substitute for heroin, but today's street dope was a lot stronger—so we'd need stronger replacement options as well. The Canadian Association of People Who Use Drugs coined the term "safe supply" to describe this concept of replacing the street drugs that were killing people with tested or pharmaceutical equivalents.

To outsiders, I was sure it would sound counterintuitive. NA would hate this idea. But I knew from years of trying that kicking dope is hard, it takes a long time, and almost everybody relapses. Even the risk of death hadn't forced me to kick. We needed a solution that would save a drug user's life right away.

For safe supply to really be effective, there could be none of the strict rules of the methadone program. No requirement to have an "opioid use disorder" diagnosis. No requirement to reduce use or quit. No piss tests. Nobody watching you take your meds. Those things would act as barriers. If this was going to work, safe supply had to be as easy as scoring street drugs. People were going to use anyway—including recreational users and weekend warriors. They needed to use something that wouldn't kill them.

Since most down was now bathtub fentanyl, I argued that doctors should prescribe pharmaceutical fentanyl instead. I had used fentanyl patches before. I knew the potency, and I was in control of the dosage. It was much safer than street dope. I wanted to fight for something that could save Laura, Chereece, Jeff . . . everybody. And if I slipped up again, I wanted it to save me too.

In November 2019, a small pilot started up to prescribe fentanyl patches. Jeff was one of the first to get on the program. He said it didn't hurt that plenty of the nurses at his clinic listened to *Crackdown* and knew he was on the editorial board. His back was soon covered in twelve plastic patches to match his large habit. His chronic pain was finally being managed, and he was feeling optimistic.

Of course we kept digging into the methadone switch too. *Crackdown* put in a Freedom of Information request to see all the emails sent between Mallinckrodt, the BC Ministry of Health and the College of Pharmacists in the lead-up to the switch. We got back reams of highly redacted government documents. Among the big black blocks of censored text, one phrase stuck out: "Exclusive Exchange Market Access Agreement." The emails revealed a secret arrangement negotiated in 2011. The BC government granted Mallinckrodt exclusive access to everyone on methadone. We were a captive market. No competition. No alternatives.

Crackdown's coverage of the switch was reported in the *Globe and Mail*. We won the Hillman Prize for Journalism, the Third Coast Festival Award for impact and a New York Festivals award. We heard that members of the provincial cabinet had listened to the episode. The former BC minister of health told me he'd called the current addictions minister to see if anything could be done. We were finally being believed.

It all put pressure on the government. Laura and I attended a meeting with provincial officials. "We could try Metadol-D," one of the officials said. It was an alternative to Methadose, a liquid version of the tablets Dr. M was prescribing me. I was shocked and angry that this had never been an option before. The government didn't give us credit, but a few months later, they made Metadol-D available to anyone who wanted it and knew to ask for it. Thousands switched off of Methadose. At long last, BCAPOM had won its demand for an alternative to Methadose that would be effective around the clock. Laura suggested we rename Metadol-D the "Chereece formulation."

Opium Ghosts

A s the drug war took more and more of my friends, I felt a need to understand how it got started. Local historian Lani Russwurm offered to take me and *Crackdown* producer Alex Kim to the place prohibition began—here, in Vancouver, not in Ottawa or Toronto. Lani had studied the secret history of this city and had an exact location in mind. If anybody could show me where prohibition began, it would be Lani.

Lani met Alex and me at Main and Hastings Streets, and we turned down the now-nameless alley behind the Carnegie Centre. A guy I knew selling rock nodded a greeting from the mouth of the alley. I smiled and shook my head, indicating that I wasn't in the market for anything. I'd been here hundreds of times, and Jeff and I used to shoot dope in this alley occasionally. It felt weird to walk in looking for history instead of looking for a fix.

We made another turn west, onto an adjoining alley that looked like so many others, with dumpsters, graffiti and oil-slick puddles. Street traffic hummed and rooftop HVACs vented dirty white noise. There were people sitting on cardboard, readying hits or leaning in alcoves, smoking rock. "Vancouver has always been the epicentre of illicit drugs in Canada," Lani said.

"It looked a lot different a century ago," he said as we walked down the narrow canyon between buildings. Back then, it was called Market Alley, he explained, and it bustled with activity, more like a main street than a place for deliveries and garbage. Actors came and went from the stage door of the Pantages Theatre, which also housed a famous boxing kangaroo, and there were restaurants, laundries and two opium factories. "This is it," Lani said, stopping in front of a doorway. "Here's where one of the city's opium factories used to operate."

I had walked past this spot a thousand times without ever noticing it.

At the turn of the twentieth century, opium and cocaine were legal. Patent medicines containing cocaine, morphine and cannabis were sold over the counter at pharmacies. You could pick up a small dark glass bottle of Bayer-brand heroin, or cocaine toothache drops or perhaps a little of Mrs. Winslow's Soothing Syrup with morphine added for good measure. Most people were free to use whatever substance they wanted—unless the person was Indigenous. The Indian Act, established soon after Confederation, contained a list of substances forbidden to "Registered Indians." The act stated, "It shall be lawful for any constable, without process of law, to arrest any Indian whom he may find in a state of intoxication." The government had long been obsessed with controlling the land, lives and bodies of Indigenous people.

There was no moral outrage about the pharmacies, but the opium dens were another story. Anti-Asian politics were sweeping North America in the early 20th century, and Vancouver was no different. Chinese, Japanese and Indian immigration was blamed for threatening the jobs and wages of white workers, as well as contributing to the growth of opium factories. Deep-seated racial prejudice was baked into mainstream politics of the day, and in August 1907, the mayor, several members of the provincial legislature and a member of Parliament formed the Vancouver chapter of the Asiatic Exclusion League. They recruited members from churches, veterans' groups and trade unions.

On Saturday, September 7, 1907, they held a big demonstration, marching along Hastings Street to an officially permitted rally at City Hall. Lani explained that at that time City Hall was located near the end of the alley. People joined as the march moved east. Banners read, "For a white Canada." Along the way, a brass band played "Rule, Britannia!" and "The Maple Leaf Forever."

A couple thousand people packed City Hall, and thousands more spilled out onto surrounding streets. Speakers whipped up the crowd. Someone lit a bonfire while others burned BC's lieutenant-governor in effigy. He had blocked a law that would've banned Asian immigration.

A young boy hurled a rock through the window of a Chinese-owned business. The sound of shattering glass touched off the riot. The white mob rampaged through Chinatown, then Market Alley, beating residents and trashing businesses as they went, including the opium factories. Rioters moved on to Powell Street, but Japanese residents had time to prepare and repelled them with sticks, rocks and bottles.

Rain eventually quelled the riot, but the news had already flashed around the world over telegraph lines. Canadian government officials were embarrassed. In the aftermath, the Asiatic Exclusion League disbanded, and Prime Minister Laurier dispatched a high-ranking official to study the damage and compensate shopkeepers for their broken windows. That official was deputy minister of labour William Lyon Mackenzie King.

Arriving in Vancouver, Mackenzie King quickly set up hearings. Businessmen, including the owners of two opium factories, appeared before him to make their claims for compensation. He approved small amounts for broken windows, damaged property and looted merchandise. But opium got his attention. Lani explained that Mackenzie King toured opium dens and reported back to Ottawa about their revenue, their workers and especially about the racial mixing of their clientele. "His concern wasn't that there were opium dens, it was that white women were using opium," Lani said.

Mackenzie King sounded the alarm, writing to Ottawa: "The habit of opium smoking was making headway, not only among white men and boys, but also among women and girls. I saw evidences of the truth of these statements in my round of visits through some of the opium dens of Vancouver." He continued: "This evil, which, once existent, does so much to destroy not only the lives of individuals, but the manhood of a nation."

Mackenzie King played into a racist myth, popular at the time, that white women were being kidnapped and forced into sexual slavery by non-white drug dealers. Historians have since debunked this idea, calling it a "moral panic." "It's the idea of fallen women," Lani said. "It was also just racism. If a white woman was associated in any way with a non-white person, she was somehow being victimized by that person."

The government passed the Opium Act in 1908. It took less than a year to go from racist riot to racist law. Emboldened by their new powers, Vancouver police started raiding opium dens. In September, they found one in Market Alley. "There were little houses," Lani said, gesturing at the doorway in front of us, where an opium den would have been. "It was probably in the basement of a house." Back in 1908, inside that basement, police caught two white women from Victoria smoking opium. The cops slapped the cuffs on the women, as well as the proprietor. One newspaper reported his name was Chun Yuen. But other papers used different names for him. It was Canada's first documented drug arrest.

Lani pulled out a pile of newspaper clippings. He pointed to the *World* newspaper's headline from 1908, which read, "Secrets of a Chinese Drug Den." Lani flipped to a *Province* headline: "In Very Basement of Their Lives: Through Trapdoor in Opium Den Detectives Discovered Two White Women Last Night."

In 1909, the government gave police more powers to search any place they considered "an opium joint" and seize what they found. In 1910–11, a cocaine panic swept Montreal, and this time Black residents were scapegoated. The panic sparked even more legislation, which banned the sale or possession of morphine and cocaine in addition to opium.

In 1922, Edmonton police magistrate and famous campaigner Emily Murphy published *The Black Candle*. Murphy wrote that the supposed foreign influence of drugs would lead to "the downfall of the white race." Upstanding citizens were becoming "ashy-faced, half-witted droolers" and "opium ghosts." Addiction, wrote Murphy, "explains the amazing phenomenon of an educated gentlewoman, reared in a refined atmosphere, consorting with the lowest classes of yellow and black men." Murphy called for harsher penalties for drug users and traffickers, immigration restrictions and racial purity. The book was not intended as a sterile policy document. It was a popular racist polemic that helped jack up fear and panic across the country. Murphy was influential in the creation of the Opium and Drug Act amendments in the 1920s, which gave the police still more powers and increased penalties for drug offences.

The RCMP had been facing cutbacks and criticism, but the drug panic gave them a whole new mission. The Mounties opened new facilities across the country, and British Columbia became Canada's drug war capital. Between 1922 and 1961, almost half of all of Canada's drug convictions occurred in BC, even though the province had less than 10 per cent of the country's population.

Mackenzie King went on to become Canada's longest-serving prime minister. Anti-Asian racism and drug panic was the fuel that drove his rise. His government passed the Chinese Exclusion Act, which banned Chinese immigration almost entirely until after World War II, during which time his government's policy on Jewish refugees fleeing the Nazis was "none is too many." He sought political advice from the spirit world, consulting mediums and attending seances in order to communicate with his departed mother and dead dog, Pat. By the mid-twentieth century, Canada was handing out some of the harshest drug penalties anywhere in the western world.

Alex packed up his microphone and we prepared to leave the alley. Lani said, "It started here, and hopefully it ends here."

"I agree," I said. "It's almost like a mandate from history that we have to end this fucking thing here."

Over a century later, the prohibition regime that was born in that alley was ready to pounce on Jeff again. He asked me to meet him at the Ovaltine Cafe on a rainy winter day. When I got there, I hung up my dripping leather jacket on the hook next to our usual booth. Grace, the owner, said hello as she put a cup of coffee down in front of me. I ordered a hot chocolate for Jeff, who rolled in a couple of minutes later and was just as wet.

"How's it going?" I asked.

"Shitty," he answered. He always said that, but today I knew it was true. Jeff's voice was raspy. It was like that when he was anxious and not sleeping enough. Jeff had another long stretch of federal time ahead of him, and his sentencing hearing was coming up. He wanted me to help him write a letter to the judge.

We ordered bacon and eggs and got down to business. The old wooden booths at the Ovaltine gave us the illusion of privacy. I poured a little Fireball Whisky from my flask into our mugs and pulled out my notebook.

The cops had busted Jeff making a couple of small deals on the street—not far from the alley Lani and I had visited. They arrested him and charged him with multiple counts of possession for the purposes of trafficking. The prosecutor was seeking years, under mandatory minimum sentencing requirements originally put in place by Stephen Harper's Conservative government.

Jeff had already done plenty of years. He would do the time if he had to, but I was worried. We were middle-aged. A long bit was harder at fifty than it was at twenty. You don't just bounce back from a shit-kicking like when you're a kid. He could lose his housing and connections to friends and the community. His medical treatment would be disrupted, and he might not even get his meds. Plus, Jeff's health wasn't great. His knee, back and neck were in constant pain. He had a serious antibiotic-resistant hospital-acquired infection. I didn't know if he'd survive. And I didn't want to be without my best friend.

I'd helped Jeff write a letter to the court before, but this would have to be our best effort yet. We needed to tell the story of Jeff's life to the judge. I had to ask him about parts of his past we'd never talked about before. I knew it was painful for him, so I treaded carefully.

I started hesitantly: "Can I ask about your mom?"

Jeff pulled out some notes he'd written and passed them across the table. "My mother gave me up for adoption when I was 8–10 months old. From what I've been able to find out, she had problems of her own. I've never met her," he'd written.

Jeff said quietly, "I guess she just threw me away." His words hung between us.

"Are you sure about that?" I asked. "Maybe your mom didn't have a choice. Maybe you were stolen by the government."

The bill of Jeff's ball cap obstructed his eyes. I felt a lump in my throat. We'd never talked about the Sixties Scoop before.

I knew Jeff would be doubtful. He never wanted to blame anyone else. He took full responsibility for the good and the bad in his life.

I looked up "Sixties Scoop" on my phone and read out the description: "An epidemic of Aboriginal child apprehension . . ." I looked over at Jeff.

Starting in the 1950s and continuing through the 1980s the government oversaw the large-scale removal of Indigenous children from their families. Tens of thousands of kids were placed into foster homes or adopted by white families. Mostly this happened without the consent of their parents or communities. The children lost their cultural identity and connections to their families and nations. Today, this policy is known as the Sixties Scoop. The law changed, but the apprehensions continue.

Jeff was quiet, processing the information. Like most people in Canada, he'd never heard of this policy. They didn't teach it in high school when Jeff and I were there.

Jeff was kidnapped, not "thrown away." Nobody ever bothered to tell him the truth. Jeff must have felt rejected and abandoned. No wonder he was a loner. How could he trust anyone after that? And no wonder he resisted authority every chance he got. The "mother's hug" of heroin must have been a lifeline for Jeff since the government denied him the real thing.

I turned to a blank page in my notebook and started drafting the story of Jeff's life for the judge. He was born on the Curve Lake First Nation in Ontario. Jeff's mother, Violet Knott, named her baby Roger. At eight months old, Roger was seized and transported to Toronto. He was adopted by the Louden family and given the name Jeff. "It's like when you get a rescue dog," Jeff said, pouring hot sauce all over his eggs, "and decide to rename it."

Jeff fondly recalled summers in Bobcaygeon with his adopted grandpa and nana. Grandpa used to buy him boxes of Cracker Jacks. One time in the forest out back of his grandparents', a moose followed Jeff. The moose must have been a year and a half old, and Jeff shared his Cracker Jacks. I could imagine how animals would have responded to Jeff's easygoing style. He's never nervous. He doesn't try to front or pretend to be anything he isn't. Jeff is just Jeff, and I'd imagine animals could tell he meant no harm. Jeff also befriended a family of owls. Then a bobcat. It was nice to relive these pleasant memories with him. He was loved and cared for.

But when school started, he had to go back to his adoptive parents' house in Scarborough. Jeff didn't really feel at home there. He said, "I was a hyper little bastard who they couldn't control anyway. And you get tired of being a punching bag." His adoptive parents insisted on a short crewcut. Kids at school teased him. He got into fights. That part sounded familiar. The Loudens returned Jeff to the foster system. It must have felt like another rejection, I thought, another abandonment.

When he was nine, another kid at a foster home offered him heroin. "You were at peace with everything," Jeff recalled. "It was like a nice little warm blanket snuggled around you."

"I bounced around in the system for a while," Jeff said. He was twelve when a social worker drove him to the home of a new foster family. They lived a long way from Toronto. It was a farm, and there was nowhere to go. Jeff was stuck there. "I had to muck out the stalls of a dozen cows, two horses, pens of rabbits and a shitload of chickens," he said. "The farmer was drunk. Every day. He carried on as though he was the smartest guy on earth. I kept my distance. I had as little to do with the farmer and his family as possible." He wasn't the only foster kid on the farm. There were five girls and two boys, plus the farmer's son. "Us foster kids ate liver and cheap cuts of meat, sloughed off in the kitchen," Jeff said. "The farmer's family supped on T-bone steak in the dining room." The food was kept under lock and key—no barrier to Jeff. The girls had a bunk room down in the basement. Jeff had to sleep in a stuffy room with the snoring grandfather.

The house was crammed with the family and a rotating cast of foster kids who came and went. The family was aloof. So was Jeff. But the land was his salvation. Outside, away from everyone except the animals, Jeff was at home. But he also had to look out for "the skinner that lived down the road." This neighbour had a predatory eye for the farm's foster kids. Jeff didn't want to talk much more about it.

Jeff spent his adolescence institutionalized. He lived in the Warrendale mental health treatment centre for children, in Etobicoke, and St. John's Training School for Boys, in Uxbridge. When I asked about this time, Jeff said, "Leave the past buried." Eventually he was sent to Camp DARE, an "alternative open-custody program for youth." Jeff described it as survival training in the woods. "I didn't want to come out of my tarp," he said. Many of these institutions have since been subject to class action lawsuits, where plaintiffs allege physical, sexual and psychological abuse. As soon as he was of age, Jeff was sent to the infamous Don Jail in Toronto, where rats would climb out the toilets, so you had to hover above the seat or risk a nasty bite in a sensitive place.

Then he was sent to the Kingston Pen, where he survived a prison riot while in hospital. Jeff spent time at Innes Road jail, near Ottawa, then Kent and Wilkinson Road jail in BC. Jeff's twenties were full of arrests for possession or petty crimes to support his drug habit. It all added up to a big chunk of Jeff's life spent incarcerated.

As we paid up, I tried to change the topic, to lighten the mood. But I could tell Jeff was tired from taking me through so many tough times. We left the Ovaltine, back into the rain.

Lisa and I wrote up the story of Jeff's life into a letter to the judge, noting Jeff's volunteer work in the community and the damage a long sentence would cause. Jeff approved the final draft. His lawyer, Sandy Ross, submitted it to the court along with a Gladue sentencing report, which reflected much of his life story. We also submitted letters from BCAPOM, VANDU and Jeff's doctor. At the hearing, the judge read out loud extensively from our letter. She was moved, and thought the prosecutor's demand that he serve years was excessive. The judge gave Jeff probation, but no custodial sentence. The system locked Indigenous people up for nonviolent drug crimes every day. But not this time. On the courthouse steps, Jeff hugged me in relief.

Disease Vectors

isa and I walked down the centre of an empty street. There were no cars. No other pedestrians. A chorus of frogs croaked in the middle of the quiet city. We were just a few blocks from our apartment, but we'd never heard them before. The pandemic had brought the world to a standstill. Governments unplugged capitalism, ordering all but essential businesses to close. But the drug war rumbled on. Unlike the overdose crisis, authorities were taking COVID seriously.

I called around to check on people. My parents, Paige, Jeff. When Jeff answered the phone, he was out on the street. I could hear the familiar soundscape of the Downtown Eastside. People were still outside while the rest of the city was bunkered in their houses.

"How's it going?" I asked Jeff.

"Shitty," Jeff said. "It's pretty pointless trying to self-isolate when you gotta share bathrooms and kitchens," he said of the single-room occupancy hotels where most people on the Downtown Eastside lived. "They're not letting any visitors in at my building," he added. Vancouver's shelters were full, which meant the city's rapidly increasing homeless population was outside too.

Crackdown producer Alex de Boer asked mayor Kennedy Stewart about it at a press conference. "There are over ten thousand Vancouverites who can't socially distance because of inadequate housing and around twenty-five thousand empty homes in the city," she said. "Will you commit to expropriating these homes to ensure Vancouver's most vulnerable residents remain safe for the coming months?" We all knew the answer, but Alex decided to ask anyway.

"No, expropriation is not on our list of things to do," Stewart responded. The city was planning to buy some old hotels, but throughout the pandemic, police would break up tent encampments and evict people to nowhere.

"VANDU's still open," Jeff said. Its injection room was running at half capacity. Vancouver's other supervised consumption sites had reduced their staff and clients as well. Yet overdose deaths were outpacing COVID deaths.

Jeff told me dealers were still working, but rock prices had spiked by a third, and down was up by 50 per cent. Crystal meth was in short supply.

A cop car rolled past Jeff. Through the phone, I heard its loudspeakers commanding, "Disperse now. Go home."

"Gotta go," Jeff said.

I called to check on Laura. "I wish I could give you a hug," she told me. Laura explained that her dealer had warned, "Get ready. Droughts are coming. You better stockpile."

"We've squirrelled a little something away," Laura said. "Are you okay?"

I told her I was. That I'd been stockpiling methadone so as not to be caught out again. I was touched that in the middle of a pandemic, Laura was checking on my supplies. She was a good friend. "Stay safe," I said, and we hung up.

My phone buzzed. It was another bad dope alert. They now came by text message from the health authority, in addition to posters on the street. "Dark purple chunks sold as down, tested positive for fentanyl and benzos and are causing severe ODs," the text read. Not only did street drugs cost more, but benzodiaze-pine-like substances—similar to Valium, Xanax and Ativan—were creeping into the drug supply. Since the summer before, I'd been seeing many overdoses involving benzos and opioids. They were worse than fentanyl alone, because naloxone only worked on the opioid part of the overdose. With benzodope, people remained unconscious—but breathing—for several hours. We had become used to that cathartic moment of revival when we brought someone back from the dead. But now they just contin-ued to lie there. Supervised consumption sites were stuffed with unconscious bodies, sleeping off benzo blackouts. A new psycho-logical burden for a community abandoned to care for itself. Fatalities started shooting up, breaking previous monthly records.

The *Crackdown* production team knew it would be a while before we'd see each other again. Like most office workers, we resorted to making the show from our separate homes. Over the next year or so, the gloomy work of documenting the overdose crisis would be done in isolation. I could feel a fog of depression settle over the whole crew. But there was also a strange feeling of opportunity in the air.

Barely a week after the world shut down, I got a call from a worried doctor who ran a Downtown Eastside clinic. She was concerned that drug users would spread COVID as they left their rooms and apartments to buy drugs. "What do drug users need in order to self-isolate? To stay quarantined?" she asked.

"Drugs," I said. "Prescribe them pharmaceutical versions of the drugs they are getting off the street." The logic was already at work. Liquor stores stayed open through the pandemic. Health officials knew that if they were shut, people would drink mouthwash or go into lethal withdrawal.

To my surprise, the doctor sounded like she was honestly considering the suggestion. I was looped into a hurried series of phone calls and text messages between doctors, government officials and academics until a new policy coalesced. Doctors would now be allowed to prescribe alternatives to street drugs. Not direct equivalents like pharmaceutical fentanyl, heroin or cocaine, but cousins—pills like Dilaudid and Ritalin. For years, the drug user movement had been calling for the real stuff because we knew it would be much more effective at reducing overdoses than weaker replacement drugs. My life had been made possible by a prescribed opioid—methadone. In the age of fentanyl, we needed stronger substitutes, and Dilaudid was a much better stand-in for street fentanyl than any formulation of methadone. As soon as the health officials could sort out the details, they promised to revise the policy to add other drugs—including prescription heroin. So this seemed like a solid first step.

I was amazed. The regular plodding pace of policy development was thrown out the window. The government's health bureaucracy was in a hurry. No one was trying to butter me up with false empathy. No crocodile tears. No endless, meaningless meetings. Just a hurried effort to write up this new plan. The final document, "Risk Mitigation in the Context of Dual Public Health Emergencies," was a rushed compromise. It made clear that it was *not* intended for treatment of "substance use disorders." Instead, the goal was to let drug users self-isolate and avoid overdose. What had been impossible for years was written and approved in a couple of weeks.

I could feel a long-dormant hope awakening in the *Crackdown* team and some of my comrades at VANDU. It was the kind of hope for a better world that had drawn us to this work in the first place. A hope that many of us had long since buried somewhere deep. We'd all become pretty good at fighting for things while telling ourselves *this probably won't work*. It was a self-protective impulse: if we expected that things would just keep getting worse, maybe it wouldn't hurt so much when they did.

"Do you think maybe COVID is going to radically transform things?" Sam asked me one day on the phone. Were we seeing the end of the drug war? I could tell by Sam's tone that he wanted to believe in what he was asking, but deep down he knew better.

"I'm sorry, man, I don't think so," I replied. "Not unless we organize and force 'em to change." Even when we were dying in huge numbers, the government was slow to respond. It was only when they started to fear us as disease vectors that they felt moved to act. I'd seen it before. The fear of us spreading HIV played the same kind of role in permitting needle programs and supervised consumption in the 1990s and early 2000s. Governments didn't care then, and they still don't care now.

There were also some serious problems with the new "risk mitigation" program. Doctors had chosen daily dosage limits to try to prevent anyone getting high off their meds. I thought about the chart Dr. M had drawn for me with the green flatline running across the centre. No euphoria. No withdrawal. That's still what the doctors wanted to achieve. But people use drugs to try to feel good. And if the doctors wanted to prevent people from getting there, I knew drug users would seek out that feeling in the deadly street supply. Just like I had.

Laura was one of the first people to get a prescription. She turned on one of *Crackdown*'s mobile recorders as she prepared her Dilaudid pills for injection. "I just hope that it's going to be a different chapter in my life," she said. I hoped so too.

The Risk Mitigation Guidance (RMG) rolled out across BC incredibly slowly. Months in, most drug users I knew still hadn't heard of the new policy. *Crackdown* offered to create a PSA for the government to run on the local rock station—which frequently blared from boom boxes and construction sites across the city. But they didn't take us up on the offer. We made our own episode anyway.

Then we started to hear that doctors were refusing to follow the guidelines. VANDU members told us that they were snapped at by the doctors when they asked for access to the program. Others said the doctor had punished them for "drug-seeking behaviour." The doctor would either reduce their other medicines or "fire them" (force them to find a new physician). My friend Hawkfeather was frightened: when they asked the doctor to consider a Dilaudid prescription, the doctor threatened to contact the child welfare system. Word got around, and many drug users became hesitant to talk to their physician about the risk mitigation meds.

Ryan McNeil filed a Freedom of Information request to try to understand why the government hadn't mandated doctors to follow the guidance. It revealed emails to the government from David Unger, deputy registrar of the College of Physicians and Surgeons. "There has been tremendous backlash on the guidelines put out thus far from doctors that manage addictions patients and addiction specialists," Unger wrote. "This should be an opportunity to engage and help these [Substance Use Disorder] patients begin the long journey to recovery as opposed to giving them drugs and just hoping they do not overdose." Unger was failing to understand our key concern. We wanted to keep people alive, and that meant giving them something to substitute for the toxic drug supply. You can't recover if you're dead.

VANDU tried its best to get the government to do something about the reluctant doctors. "Would you allow the doctors to disobey COVID guidelines?" I asked on one Zoom call. Why was providing good overdose prevention care *optional* when other health practices were mandatory? But the flurry of policy making energy that we'd experienced at the start of the pandemic had died off. We began to get the sense that many inside the BC NDP—particularly premier John Horgan and minister of health Adrian Dix—now viewed the risk mitigation program as a political liability. Whenever possible, Horgan and Dix avoided discussing it—as well as the overdose crisis—in public.

One exception was BC's chief coroner, Lisa Lapointe. She continued to champion the policy and called out those that refused to implement it. "There are very many [doctors] who are reluctant because they don't agree with prescribing drugs that people very often are addicted to," she told journalist Ian Mulgrew. "They see it as a harm. The colleges are not supportive and no one wants . . . the college [to] come look over their shoulder at what they're doing." Lisa Lapointe had seen the bodies stacking up. She'd counted them every month. She'd reviewed every possible intervention, and she knew that prescribing alternatives was the most effective way to get someone to avoid using street drugs. She seemed frustrated that the health care system was too timid to make it happen.

In the first year of the pandemic, fatal overdoses increased dramatically. More people were dying of overdose than of COVID, motor vehicle accidents, murder and suicide combined. Benzodope had made things so much worse. Laura wasn't at BCAPOM meetings as much. Her Dilaudid prescription just wasn't enough, and benzodope had her blacked out for hours. I missed her. When we saw each other, we'd talk and I'd try to help sort things out. But the next time I saw her, she couldn't remember. I felt like I was losing my friend three hours or three days at a time.

If heroin was a warm blanket, then fentanyl was a thunder blanket. But benzodope could be like getting buried alive. It sounds extreme, but I understood. Sometimes you just needed to hit the off switch. I had used prescription opioids and benzos together to give myself a guaranteed dreamless sleep. But benzodope was creating chaos. The overdoses were worse, and trying to kick could give you fatal seizures. Detox had become complicated and dangerous.

VANDU meetings devolved into a jumble of mumbling voices talking over each other and off topic. The meetings used to be tight. We used to come to order right on the hour. We had an agenda, and the chair would keep us on track. Our sergeant-at-arms would keep order, and the membership itself would silence interruptions and remind each other to keep on topic. Not anymore. It had all come apart. People had to blurt out their thoughts or risk forgetting them. Nobody could recall what had been discussed the previous week—or even what had been discussed during the previous agenda item.

Benzodope didn't look fun. Some people were bent over at nearly a right angle, facing the floor, as if the hinge at their waist could no longer open all the way. Drug users are not known for our military-straight postures, but I never used to see people walking down Hastings folded in half like a jack-knife, or standing still, contorted like a pretzel. A benzo black-out could leave you doubled over for hours, and even when you woke up, your back was still bent. After enough days and weeks of that, your posture changed. There were a lot more people using wheelchairs, scooters and walkers. Those black-outs would slowly eat away at your memories and histories. There'd be missing pages in the story of your life. More and more pages until the plot didn't make sense, until it seemed like a different book. You'd wake up, hours later, missing your dope, phone or wallet because someone had been digging through your pockets. Some women woke up to discover they had been sexually assaulted during the blackout.

Familiar faces looked at me from memorial posters on lampposts. Sometimes of an acquaintance I'd seen around the place for years but never gotten the opportunity to really know. Other times, of close friends and comrades. *Crackdown* editorial board member Dave Murray died, not of an overdose but of septicemia. Dave was a neighbourhood intellectual with taped glasses and a newspaper always tucked under his arm.

VANDU was struggling to hold memorials for every member individually. Instead, we had to hold a mass funeral—a grim first. I was responsible for eulogizing three people.

Amidst all the death, it became clear that the government no longer intended to add prescription heroin or other potentially life-saving medicines to its risk mitigation program. The scientific consensus on COVID-19 was changing, and the policy makers no longer saw drug users scoring drugs outside as much of a threat. To politicians, the risk mitigation policy was a political liability. We started to hear rumblings from sources inside the BC NDP government. They were considering jettisoning the program, even as deaths from the toxic street supply continued to increase. At its height, the risk mitigation program reached around five thousand people. That's only about 2 per cent of the drug users across BC.

Any faint hope we had in government programs had evaporated. If we wanted a safe supply, we were going to have to do it ourselves.

Safe Supply or We Die

They're giving free drugs out over there," said a guy on the street.

"Yeah right," his buddy replied, barely breaking his stride. They were out of earshot before anyone had the chance to tell him, "No, seriously! We actually are!"

The crowd kept growing until it filled VANDU and spilled onto the sidewalk. "It's probably a good thing people think this is too good to be true," I said to Jeff. "Otherwise we'd have thousands trampling in here."

It was a sunny day. My albinism had trained me to think of the sun as a kind of enemy, so I stood in shade when I could and wore a big black cowboy hat. I figured if Johnny Winter could make it look cool, maybe I could pull it off too. I could tell that the nice weather was lifting everyone's spirits. I was buoyed along by their energy. "This is a good day," I said to Jeff.

"If your name's not on this list, you won't get any drugs!" Pockets' voice boomed over the hubbub of the crowd. Pockets—VANDU's six-foot-two, barrel-chested sergeant-at-arms—had no difficulty making himself heard above the noise. Over the years, Pockets had demonstrated an uncanny ability to control chaotic situations, de-escalate tension, and move people along—all with such earnest friendliness that people mostly didn't mind. But this job—deciding who would and wouldn't get free drugs—seemed like a tall order even for him. I noticed that his *Taxi Driver* T-shirt was already soaked in sweat.

Pockets asked the crowd to shout out their names, one by one, and he frantically scribbled each name down on his clipboard, making sure he recognized everyone on the list. "Only seasoned vets, no kids, no first-timers," he reminded the crowd. Then he started handing out green wristbands.

I got a wristband too. I wasn't planning on doing any of these drugs myself. But I figured I should at least grab some for Jeff. Mostly, I just wanted to hang with my friends and be a part of the historic occasion.

A journalist asked me, "How could any drug be safe?"

"We never know the purity or potency of street dope," I answered. "Your hit could be 50 per cent fentanyl or 0 per cent. It could contain industrial cleansers, rat poison, pig dewormer, cement, brick dust or baby laxative. Not knowing is what'll kill you. The coroner says that's why thousands of people are dying. The Drug User Liberation Front tests the drugs so potency and purity are assured. It's a little example of how the government could regulate the drug market, like it does with coffee, tobacco and booze. Nothing is 100 per cent safe, but a regulated supply would end this crisis."

The idea had started months earlier. May 2020 was the deadliest month we'd seen in the crisis yet. Then June became the deadliest month. Then July. It seemed like every month would come with a new, grim record. So a group of activists representing various organizations called an emergency Zoom meeting to discuss what to do next.

The meeting began the way most of our meetings went around that time. We caught each other up on who had died since we last spoke, and we vented our rage about government inaction. Why hadn't they stepped up the risk mitigation program? Why weren't they doing anything? Then someone said, "Well, what are we going to do about it?"

Ann Livingston reminded us of our movement's history of civil disobedience. In the 1990s, activists didn't wait around for the government to grant them permission to distribute syringes or open a supervised consumption site. They took direct action. Because some things are more important than following the law. And because, they figured, if the cops and courts had the guts to try to prosecute them, they'd have a decent shot at winning a Charter challenge. After all, they were saving lives.

"We need to do the same thing for safe supply," we all agreed. The plan flowed out of the group with ease, like we'd all been dreaming of this for ages. We would give away free, tested heroin, meth and cocaine. We knew we'd never be able to get enough drugs together to actually replace the whole contaminated street supply. But our giveaway could provide some drug users with a temporary refuge from deadly illicit drugs while serving as a brazen challenge to the government.

This was in no way a new idea. In the early 1950s, the Community Chest and Council of Greater Vancouver—a charity somewhat like the United Way—appointed a special committee on narcotics and produced the Ranta Report. It recommended changing federal drug laws so that narcotics clinics could be established where drug users could get "their minimum required dosages." Newspapers reprinted the whole report and endorsed it in editorials. In the 2000s, the North American Opiate Medication Initiative (NAOMI) and the Study to Assess Long-term Opioid Medication Effectiveness (SALOME) both showed the huge benefits of prescription heroin. In all cases, the government ignored the expert advice, opting to continue the punitive drug war instead. I sometimes imagined the alternative futures we would have if the government had listened. Fentanyl might not have happened. China White might not have happened. A hundred or so people I knew as friends and acquaintances might still be here.

We didn't want any existing group to take on the legal risks, so we decided to form a new group with a new name. Harkening back to the militancy of sixties and seventies radicals, we called ourselves the Drug User Liberation Front, or DULF, and began planning our first action.

Right away, we ran into a big problem: where to get clean drugs? As the police continued to bust dealers and tighten up the borders, the illicit drug market innovated. Suppliers started selling more and more potent kinds of dope—carfentanil, benzodope or tranqdope with livestock sedatives. These were easier to hide from the cops. We didn't want any of this crap in the drugs we gave away, but so far, Health Canada had not granted us legal standing to buy from pharmaceutical companies. So several DULF members called the most trustworthy dealers they knew. For weeks, DULF activists scoured the suburbs, scoring dope in parking lots in Abbotsford and Chilliwack. Our first batch tested positive for fentanyl, so we couldn't give it out. Trying to source drugs was time-consuming, frustrating and risky.

I thought maybe we should keep some of DULF's activities on the down low. Ideally, anyone involved in sourcing the drugs should be known to as few people as possible. It would be less of a heat score. But two of the most energetic activists in our group, Eris Nyx and Jeremy Kalicum, took the lead. They became DULF's main spokespeople to the media. Eris and Jeremy were perfect, in part because of their captivating, odd-couple dynamic.

Eris was a trans punk drug user and the singer for a local band called Dust Blaster. She often wore a black beret, army boots and camouflage fatigues to show that we were in a war. She had a no-bullshit way of talking that rang out through a megaphone or a TV camera. "We're always afraid of getting arrested, but I've also always done drugs," Eris said in an interview for *Crackdown*. "And if the drugs are safe, and the drugs are good, I feel better about doing that than not knowing what the fuck I've got my hands on."

Jeremy, by comparison, came off much more straight-laced and reserved. "I'm a complete square," he told me. "I had never even tried, or really *seen*, many drugs." Instead, Jeremy explained that he'd grown up working class and was desperate to get a legitimate career. He'd discovered the drug user movement while doing volunteer work that he hoped would give him an edge when applying to med school. Through that work, he learned to love the pragmatic compassion of harm reduction. He became good friends with many drug users, and he was radicalized by all the death.

DULF decided to stop trying to source drugs from local suppliers and look for clean dope on the dark web instead, gradually developing and refining a complex process that wouldn't leave a trail for the cops. The first step was to raise the group's public profile by doing as many media hits as possible, organizing benefit concerts and shouting about our plans at rallies. Then we used our growing notoriety to raise money from donors, which was converted into Bitcoin and then exchanged for Monero (an untraceable cryptocurrency). Using a computer running Linux and Tor Browser, DULF accessed dark web markets where vendors sold drugs. The cryptocurrency was held in escrow until the drugs arrived in the mail, and we tested them with Fourier-transform infrared spectrometry. If they passed the test, the drugs were packaged into small hits that contained potency information and warning labels. The plan worked.

I admired Eris and Jeremy's bravery, but also worried that they were taking on a lot of personal risk. They both acted like it was no big deal, but deep down we all knew what the stakes were.

It was finally time for the DULF giveaway to start. VANDU activists closed off the 300 block of East Hastings to make space for the celebration. Instead of traffic, the six-lane street was full of Downtown Eastside residents, harm reduction workers, drug users, artists, musicians, activists and journalists. Among the sea of signs and placards, one banner quoted a NOFX lyric: "The only drug problem is scoring real good drugs."

At the front of the party, a guitarist with a local band called Bedwetters Anonymous ripped into the opening chords of

AC/DC's "Thunderstruck." Young punks, Indigenous grandmas and street nurses got on their feet and danced in the sun. The sound of classic rock covers filled the air. On a bad day, Sam and I could both be a little snobby about music, but as the drummer launched into an epic fill, Sam smiled and said, "I like this tune."

"Me too," I replied.

"How about some Megadeth," Jeff mumbled. But I knew he was a sucker for old AC/DC.

I was hungry, so I walked to the barbecue, where my friend Makeda Martin was turning hot dogs and hamburgers on a massive grill. "No charge," she said. It wasn't just the drugs that were free today—it was the burgers too. I gladly took some food, remembering that Makeda's niece Regis had been killed when the Toronto Police were doing a wellness check. Instead of letting her grief and rage destroy her, Makeda poured herself into feeding the community, opening a free kitchen and distributing food boxes throughout the pandemic. I thanked her for the hot dog and decided to check out some of the nearby stalls.

My first stop was to a booth where *Crackdown* editorial board newcomer Reija Jean was reading tarot cards.

"Sit down," she told me, "and pick out two cards." I pulled the Ten of Swords and the Ten of Pentacles but managed to reverse them when putting them down. "Hmm," Reija said. "You've kinda mixed up the meaning by doing that." I had no idea what these cards meant, but somehow I'd screwed it up. Jeff snorted.

"I guess I'm fucking up my future again," I quipped. Reija rolled her eyes and laughed politely.

"How ya doing, dove?" said a friendly voice out of the blue. "We're giving away donuts!" It was the anti-racist activist and musician Tonye Aganaba. Tonye was part of a coalition—the Defund 604 Network—that wanted to reduce the Vancouver Police Department budget and invest in the community instead. "The donuts are just a little joke," Tonye said. I wondered if the dozens of cops lurking around the edges of our party felt tempted by the baked goods.

Eris was on the mic, presiding over the whole thing like a ringmaster at a circus. Today she wasn't in her usual military garb, instead opting for a Willy Wonka costume. It was part of a *Charlie and the Chocolate Factory* theme that I didn't totally understand.

"I don't know, I was drunk when I thought it up," Eris laughed.

Either way, I thought, the outfit matched the mood. Eris proceeded to emcee the carnival. She called up Jean Swanson, Vancouver's veteran anti-poverty organizer and city councillor, who was now in her seventies. Jean produced three white boxes with a black flame logo that were clearly labelled "Heroin," "Cocaine" and "Methamphetamine." She then handed the boxes to Pockets so that he could distribute their contents to drug users. Unbeknownst to the assembled cops, the boxes were empty. None of us *actually* wanted to risk Jean's arrest. But the political theatre was clear. "If you're gonna arrest the activists, well then you'd better be willing to arrest me as well."

Jeff and I headed back to VANDU, where Pockets had set up a table in the doorway, and VANDU members with wristbands lined up to get the drugs. In his booming voice, Pockets called our names one by one. A few random people attempted to cut in line, but Pockets pleasantly waved them off, repeating over and over, "No wristband, no dope."

"Garth!" Pockets said, as I reached the front of the line. "Heroin, coke or meth?"

"Heroin," I said. Pockets handed me a little white box. I looked at the packaging. It read, "diacetylmorphine [heroin]— 96.5%, morphine—1.4%, codeine—2.1%." In big letters the package also read, "CAUTION: keep away from children or pets" and "WARNING: this product contains heroin which is a highly addictive substance." Inside were two tiny plastic envelopes, each holding one-tenth of a gram of beige powder. This wouldn't be enough to get anyone around here high, but it made the point.

Damn, I thought. This wasn't orange sand, green crystals or purple pebbles. This was old-school heroin. As I held the package in my hand, it felt like the culmination of a decades-long dream. The fulfillment of the policy solution that we had been championing for ages.

This is how we stop the dying, I thought, as the block party raged behind me.

"Here, take this," I said to Jeff, handing him my two points of heroin. "If it's on me much longer, I'm likely to use it."

Jeff happily obliged.

DULF's stunt was big news. Suddenly Eris and Jeremy were everywhere: in the newspaper, on local TV news, and in *Time* magazine. But the cops and government stood down. DULF held a couple more big giveaway events and started a smaller "Dope On Arrival" program. Each month, when the coroner released her latest overdose fatality statistics, DULF would give out tested drugs to a few dozen community members at VANDU. The group had been waiting to hear back on our request for an exception to the Controlled Drugs and Substances Act, which would make the giveaways legal and would allow us to source the drugs from a pharmaceutical manufacturer. When Health Canada rejected the application, DULF got a lawyer and filed a judicial review.

DULF remained undeterred. The giveaway events were fun, powerful demonstrations of the kinds of programs that were possible. But we all recognized the quantities we were handing out wouldn't make a big difference in people's lives. Most of the recipients would likely have to use street dope again later that day. And so the group decided to create an unsanctioned compassion club. DULF put out a call for applicants to join the new club and then selected forty-seven through a lottery system. Each of them could buy—at cost—whatever amount of tested heroin, coke or meth they needed on a given day. And they could use their drugs at a supervised consumption site operated by DULF. Within a year, the compassion club had significantly reduced hospitalizations, drug-related violence, negative interactions with police, and overdoses amongst its membership. DULF was no longer just organizing symbolic actions: we were showing on a small scale what was possible.

But I knew that we wouldn't be able to stop the mass dying ourselves. There were 225,000 people at risk of overdose in BC, and we were using all of our resources to help just forty-seven of them. DULF couldn't replace the prescribing capacity of the government's health system. But our compassion club showed what the federal and provincial governments could have been doing all along. *They* had the power to do what DULF did, but on a big scale. They could regulate drugs.

Being part of the solution made things feel a little less bleak. DULF was showing the world that the overdose crisis wasn't an intractable problem befuddling our smartest policy makers and scientists. It could be solved. But only if our elected officials had the courage to act. That's probably why they decided to take us down.

Backlash

Stumbles was the first one to detect the tiny heartbeat. Purring, our little cat curled up on Lisa's stomach in bed at night—staying as close as possible to her for the next several days. At first we didn't understand why.

Lisa and I had been trying to have kids for a few years, and we'd learned to temper our expectations. Maybe it was too late. I could tell how badly Lisa wanted to be a mom, and I knew that she'd be great at it. I wondered if she'd be okay if it ended up just being the two of us.

The truth was, I blamed myself for our situation. Maybe I'd just taken too long to get my shit together. For years, I felt like I'd be doing the world a favour by not having kids. I thought it would be irresponsible to pass my addict and albino genes down to a new generation.

That all changed when I met Lisa, got PTSD treatment and started to work through the stuff that happened with Victoria. I often looked after Paige. And I found that I had a knack for it. I was letting go of the shame about my albinism and drug use too. I was reaching middle age—but I finally felt like I was in the right place to become a parent. I put my hand on Lisa's stomach.

"I'd be okay if the baby has albinism," Lisa said, reading my mind. "I'd be happy."

Over the next few weeks, the embryo grew from the size of a sweet pea to a blueberry. Lisa and I were still *officially* setting realistic expectations and not getting ahead of ourselves. But deep down I could tell we were dreaming of our new future. Lisa said I should quit smoking, and I finished my last pack. We started talking about baby names. We got on waiting lists for daycare. I even started to ask my co-workers if I could have their old high chairs and cribs.

"I can't wait to meet the little ankle biter," Jeff said. And Dean pulled me aside after a *Crackdown* editorial board meeting to give me advice on fatherhood. We had become good friends. It felt like everyone around VANDU was excited. The idea of a new life offered a little hope amidst all the death and misery of the drug war.

I was excited too. But from time to time I'd also feel a wave of fear. What if the government fucked up the methadone program again? What if I relapsed? What if I couldn't take the pressure of fatherhood? It had taken me so long to build my life to this point. Was I ready to stress-test it with an infant? *Junkie, ghost, freak, loser, fuck-up*. I'd learned to turn the self-hating voice in my head down to a whisper. But it was still there. And I struggled to put my feelings into words with Lisa. I wondered if she could sense my fear.

Then one night Lisa woke up to Stumbles pawing at her insistently. "I feel a fluttering," she said to me. And then suddenly Lisa felt nothing. A few anxious days later she was curled up on the bathroom floor, convulsing in agony. I sat with her throughout the long night while Stumbles stood guard with a worried look on her little cat face. We were losing the baby. The next day, I collected our cancelled future in a small specimen jar. The lab told us it would've been a girl.

A black cloud descended over us. I supported Lisa, but I could see her hope for the future fade. I floated on an ocean of guilt. I felt ashamed to have ever worried about fatherhood. It would have been an honour to be a dad. I had helped raise Paige and she had grown into a smart, kind and musically gifted young person. At workplace gatherings, people handed me their fussy babies and they'd calm down. I realized that I'd been ready to be a dad for years.

Lisa and I cried together in bed. I was worried about her, about the deep hole she was falling into. I tried to apologize, but the words got stuck in my throat. I knew she'd tell me that this wasn't my fault and that she loved me. But I was committed to punishing myself for this loss.

Over the next several grief-grey months, I couldn't stop, I had to keep moving, keep going. I was there for Lisa as she mourned the miscarriage. But other than that I was only going through the motions of ordinary life. I worked my union job. I kept up a weekly cycle of meetings and organizing at VANDU. I struggled to come up with anything to say in *Crackdown*'s scripts. The show now had a pretty large listenership. Every week, I got messages from other drug users thanking me for the way I portrayed myself and for helping them see that we didn't have to hate ourselves. *But I do hate myself*, I thought. "Thanks for the kind words," I responded.

I was pretty sure Sam and Alex de Boer were scratching their heads, looking at the lacklustre writing I'd done on our scripts. I tried to dig down and find a way to fake the kind of strident self-assuredness that had become *Crackdown*'s voice. *I have to keep it together for the sake of the listeners and the movement*, I thought. But more and more often, Sam and Alex would just fix the writing themselves. Looking back, it would have been better to just come clean. I was in trouble.

The next several months were bleak. I learned to open Facebook only when I was braced for bad news. One day, I read that an old friend from the punk scene had died of an overdose. Janis's body was discovered outside of a Toronto supervised consumption site, but it was closed at the time of her death. She'd still be alive if the site had been open. In the summer of 2024, the Ontario government would announce that the site would close forever, along with more than half of the supervised consumption sites in the province, thus ensuring many more such tragedies.

When my pal Wade Crawford died, I was relieved to learn it hadn't been an overdose. I still don't know why that mattered to me. In 1991, Wade had stood against developers who wanted to expand a golf course on Kanehsatake, including on an Indigenous burial site. Wade and his comrades formed a blockade of the Mercier Bridge and held their ground for over a month as the Canadian Army laid siege. The newspapers called it the Oka Crisis. At Wade's memorial, VANDU members filled a notebook with stories about what a great friend and valued community member he was. I sent the notebook to his dad in Six Nations.

Soon Lisa was pregnant again—but this time we knew better than to let ourselves dream of the future. I'm not sure how much that helped. When we lost that pregnancy too, we were gutted. Lisa's mom was then diagnosed with a terminal brain disease. Through tears, Lisa told me, "I feel like there's nothing to look forward to." It was too much. Everything in our lives was dying. I felt like I was drowning. And I pushed the grief down.

After more than ten years sticking only to methadone, I wanted the old relief of heroin. I *needed* it. I didn't want street dope, so I started to buy Dilaudid and other prescription opioids off friends. I kept my new drug use hidden from Lisa. "You gotta tell her," Jeff said. I knew he was right. "I just don't want to put one more problem on her plate," I said. And I didn't say anything. I worried she'd leave me if she thought I was falling back into old habits.

"It's really sad that in this war on drug users, in this war on the poor, that we have to keep doing these memorials," organizer Vince Tao told me and the other mourners gathered at VANDU. "But this is at the heart of what VANDU does."

It was April 2022, and *Crackdown* editorial board member Greg Fresz had recently died. Greg had been a local hockey star in New Westminster. He was a member of a patients' rights group called the SALOME/NAOMI Association of Patients that many had credited with saving the city's small prescription heroin program.

"When people die at VANDU," Vince continued, "you're still a member." And then, repeating himself for emphasis:

"You're *always* a member." The room nodded along with Vince's preacherly pace and delivery.

"And that's because for the revolutionary, death is not the end," Vince said. "We have to continue Greg's work. We must! Because we mourn the dead, but we fight for the living!" A small cheer came from the crowd. The lethargy in the room was being replaced with inspiration.

"Every single time we mourn one of our past soldiers, one of our past warriors, one of our past leaders," Vince said, "it's also a challenge to us to make sure there is not one more. Is that right, folks?"

"Hell yeah!" someone shouted from the crowd, and everyone cheered. I remembered Nick's funeral. This couldn't have been more different. *This is how we should always remember our friends and family when they die*, I thought.

Vince called us all to stand for a moment of silence. He told us that he knew it felt like we were at the bottom. That many of us felt like we couldn't possibly keep fighting. But that we must keep fighting. Because our opponents were just starting to get organized.

I threw myself into work for the movement. At the time, the BC government seemed open to decriminalizing the personal possession of small amounts of heroin, cocaine and methamphetamine—something the drug user movement had pushed for since its inception. I knew it was important for VANDU to be involved in the conversations around how decriminalization would be structured in BC. In 2019, I had gone to Portugal with Lisa and Sam to make a *Crackdown* episode about the decriminalization model there. We went to a shooting gallery on the outskirts of Porto with Rui Miguel, a board member of Portugal's drug user union. While there, the cops raided the neighbourhood, chasing after drug dealers. "But aren't drugs decriminalized here?" we asked. Rui explained that Portuguese decriminalization was an unfinished revolution. You wouldn't go to jail for less than a gram, but drugs were still illegal and the police still busted people. As we packed up to leave, Rui gave me a piece of comradely advice: if governments in Canada ever set out to decriminalize drugs, "make sure you're in the room."

VANDU learned that provincial officials were going to be discussing decriminalization at a series of Core Planning Table meetings, to be held regularly over Zoom. VANDU's board decided to send me and our executive director, Brittany Graham. We knew that the discussions would get into the minutiae of the law, so we asked Pivot Legal Society lawyer Caitlin Shane to back us up. Many friends of our organization would be there too, including drug user activists from rural BC and representatives from Moms Stop the Harm—a group of parents who'd lost kids to overdose. Then there would be groups that we felt we would have common cause with, including health researchers and organizations like the First Nations Health Authority. And of course there would be cops. The meetings to decide how to remove police from our lives would feature Vancouver Police and RCMP brass as well as a representative from the Canadian Association of Chiefs of Police. We knew the cops would be pushing for a form of decrim where they would still have the most power over our lives. Our job was to make sure they didn't win.

At the first meeting, I took the floor to explain the drug user movement's vision. I said that decrim had originated as a demand from our movement. It meant that the police should simply stop apprehending people possessing drugs. No more carding. No more stop-and-search. No more seizing drugs, paraphernalia or cash. No more violence and harassment. No more handcuffs or submission holds. No more arrests, courts, jails and red zones. No more ankle monitors, probation officers and piss tests. No more child apprehensions, evictions or firings simply by virtue of a possession charge. All of this stuff just pushes us into the alleys and shadows, where we are more likely to use alone and die. And all of that policing had never stopped drugs anyway.

The police sat and listened on Zoom—some in uniform and others in golf shirts. These weren't beat cops. They were the top brass, slick and trained in communications. For the good of appearances, they acted like we were friends, even though they'd been locking us up since 1908. Brittany and I built a consensus among everyone else that possession thresholds should be set according to the quantity of drugs that users would need over a three-day period. We had plenty of data from a survey of VANDU members to back us up. But the major elements of the policy were set by politicians and senior officials behind closed doors.

In January 2023, I crunched through new-fallen snow while recording myself on my phone. BC's decriminalization pilot had just begun. It was now legal for anyone over nineteen to carry up to 2.5 grams total of opioids, cocaine, meth or MDMA. If you were caught, it wouldn't be seized and you wouldn't be jailed, fined or otherwise punished. "And—let's see what I've got here," I said—talking to the *Crackdown* producers and listeners I imagined might eventually hear me. "Just about, like, I'd say a half gram—a half gram of, you know, 90 per cent pure heroin. Old-school, tan-coloured heroin. And, um . . . technically I'm a perfect law-abiding citizen right now!" It felt historic. I tried to hold on to the feeling of victory. But as I walked, my optimism started to melt into slush. This could never last. The political winds were changing.

I'd started worrying about the backlash in January 2022. *They're going to come for us next,* I thought as I watched the news. Images of hundreds of trucks, a right-wing convoy, flickered on the screen. The vehicles—along with thousands of protesters—had converged on Ottawa and occupied the blocks around Parliament Hill. Canada's burgeoning right-wing populist movement was against masks and vaccine mandates for the time being. But bubbling underneath was Alberta separatism, anti-trans bigotry and white supremacist anti-immigration politics. The convoy had a plan to replace the government—and it seemed like it could work.

The news report showed a number of mainstream conservative politicians greeting the convoy. They stood in their suits and ties, taking selfies with the protesters and handing out donuts. The right had found one another and united. How long before they found us?

For decades, Canadian politics had been bogged down in a kind of mushy complacency. Successive Conservative and Liberal regimes tweaked the country a few degrees to the right or to the centre—mostly maintaining the increasingly untenable status quo. It didn't matter that climate emergencies were now nearly constant. It didn't matter that more and more people couldn't afford a home (even people who had good jobs). It didn't matter that every major urban centre now had a tent encampment. Or that grocery barons had been fixing the price of bread. Or that people were dying in droves from contaminated drugs. It didn't matter that police budgets were out of control. It didn't matter that the health system was crumbling and that mental health care was out of reach for most. Our elected officials had commitments to industry, capital and ideology that stopped them from taking real action on the escalating crises all around us. Perhaps the state had cut itself back so much since the time of Reagan and Thatcher that they really were powerless—at least powerless to do anything good.

I had spent my lifetime in movements that put forward bold plans to solve the challenges around us: tax the billionaires, expropriate empty homes, redistribute wealth hoarded at the very top, unionize the workforce, give the land back to the Indigenous nations who owned it, transition off of fossil fuels, cut police budgets, invest in communities and end the drug war. The government had never tried any of it, spending more effort opposing or co-opting us. But over the years, squishy neo-liberals—including the leaders of the BC NDP and the federal Liberal Party—had frequently branded their tiny pilot projects and incremental actions using our words and concepts. Never big or bold enough to address the actual problems, these anemic half measures became ideal propaganda targets for Canada's resurgent right wing. They argued that these "woke" policies were the cause of the mess, rather than potential solutions, albeit on a microscopic scale.

Later that fall, in the run-up to Vancouver's mayoral election, several right-wing candidates ran on law-and-order platforms. Gesturing at all of the genuine social suffering around him, Ken Sim argued that Vancouver had become a dangerous, drug-infested hellscape. Sim's answer was more cops. He promised that, if elected, he would immediately hire one hundred more police officers. Soon, Sim had the endorsement of the police union. He won in a landslide. Sim and the police were part of an ascendant political wave that was just getting started. Nothing changed except taxes went up to pay for all the new cops.

In November, Pierre Poilievre, the leader of the federal Conservative Party, released a video called "Everything Feels Broken." The video, shot in CRAB Park on Vancouver's waterfront, featured a tent encampment as set decoration. Poilievre blamed the homelessness behind him on one single thing: drugs. On the video, he never bothered to talk to any of the campers. A huge amount of overdose deaths were occurring among men in the trades at the time. The toxic drug supply was killing people from every walk of life, not just homeless people. Poilievre didn't blame toxic street drugs; he specifically blamed BC's tiny risk mitigation prescribing program.

"This is a deliberate policy by woke Liberal and NDP governments," Poilievre said, "to provide taxpayer-funded drugs—flood our streets with easy access to these poisons. This has been tried . . . and always with the same results: major increases in overdoses and a massive increase in crime."

"Everything Feels Broken" instantly struck me as a political winner. Everything *did* feel broken. And Poilievre's major political rival, Justin Trudeau, would be hard-pressed to argue that it didn't. Poilievre's video was total bullshit, but I knew that wouldn't matter. The idea that the BC NDP's tiny risk mitigation program was *responsible* for overdose death was laughably easy to disprove. The program came along *six years* into the overdose crisis. And coroners' data showed that the government's Dilaudid prescriptions had not caused a single overdose fatality. It didn't matter that Poilievre called the program a "flood" when, at its peak, Dillies had only trickled out to 2 per cent of drug users.

The political centre—the federal Liberal Party and the BC NDP—unwilling to pursue bold policy change, now found themselves in an unenviable position: to stay in power, they needed to convince voters that things weren't as bad as they seemed. And I knew Poilievre would gain thousands of fans simply by acknowledging that the housing and overdose crisis were, in fact, serious and unacceptable problems. Not to mention, Poilievre's conspiracy theory was just too juicy to ignore—the idea that the drug user movement had fought for a program that was responsible for our deaths. And "Everything Feels Broken" shot up to hundreds of thousands of views.

While I grew up on the left, Poilievre was coming of age in the campus clubs of Canada's conservative movement. While I was protesting the right-wing populist Reform Party, Poilievre was working in its leader's office. While I marched to defend Canada's only supervised consumption site, Poilievre held several cabinet posts in the Conservative government of Stephen

Harper, who was trying to shut it down. Unlike most other politicians, Poilievre understood the power of a movement. He's a lifelong movement conservative, true believer and free-market fundamentalist.

Before long, Poilievre had figured out that campaigning on our corpses was a political winner. We became one of the central planks of his polemics against Trudeau. Across the country, municipal and provincial politicians learned the same lesson and stepped up their fearmongering about the country's "lawlessness" and "disorder." The world was tired of hearing about our problems, and they wanted someone authoritative to make us go away. Poilievre promised to end decriminalization and defund safe supply when he takes office. He promised to close supervised consumption sites—calling them "drug dens"—an echo of the opium moral panics at the dawn of Canada's drug war. As this book goes to print, Poilievre looks set to become Canada's next prime minister.

I did my best to raise the alarm among VANDU's membership— many of whom didn't have access to televised news or the internet. We held a large general meeting, where we outlined the major figures in the ascendant right-wing campaign against us. VANDU members booed when they watched video of Poilievre and his colleagues in the House of Commons. "How can he be so out of touch?" one member asked. Others couldn't help but laugh as Poilievre described drug use awkwardly.

"I'd take him seriously, though," I cautioned. "This guy wants to tear down everything we've fought for."

———

BC's premier, John Horgan, retired and was replaced by David Eby. I'd known Eby years earlier when he was a lawyer for Pivot, representing poor people on the Downtown Eastside. He now seemed keen to prove to the world that those days were long behind him. Eby had been musing about forcing people into treatment and reopening Riverview, a creepy Edwardian mental hospital, long since closed. Other politicians, like BC Conservative Party leader John Rustad, had their own version of the same plan. If forced treatment had been the law when I was using heroin, I would never have tried to get on the methadone program, out of fear of getting locked up. I would never have been able to trust the doctor. If I was forced into treatment, I would try to escape. Once I got out, I would want to use for sure, but my tolerance might be lowered, thus making me more vulnerable to overdose. If I overdosed, a friend might be reluctant to call 911, worried that I'd get hauled off. The lives of drug users have already been stripped of so much self-determination. Stripping away our rights wouldn't stop the deaths—it would increase them.

In January 2023, Global News ran a province-wide televised news story about prescribed Dilaudid. "Those working in the recovery sector say kids aged sixteen and seventeen are getting their hands on those drugs," the newscaster said, citing no evidence apart from a single interview with the director of a recovery facility. It was frustrating. It was so much easier to scare people with a simple story than explain the nuances of reality. But the truth doesn't matter when the spectre of kids using drugs is raised.

The first place most kids access pills is a family member's medicine cabinet. Dilaudid and other pills have been available and accessible to youth since I was one. When prescription pills become less available, pill-pressed fakes fill the gap and often contain fentanyl. These are more likely to be instantly fatal. The mere availability of something isn't what causes people to get wired. Nobody wants a young person to use a substance that will harm them. But youth use drugs, and this isn't new. Even in the 1980s, as a teen, I knew where to get drugs. Alcohol, pills, coke, heroin, meth—all were accessible in some form or another. Now, the internet makes buying anything as simple as a few clicks. Generations brought up online know where to get substances. It might be news to adults that kids do drugs and know where to get them, but no one who really listens to young people would be surprised. Kids need real drug education—not the DARE-like programming I got, which is still all too common today. But if a teenager is hell-bent on experimenting with opioids, they're much, much more likely to find lethal street fentanyl than a Dilaudid tablet. The coroner tells us that it is street fentanyl, not Dilaudid, that's causing the mass deaths. The Global news story didn't provide viewers with any of this context.

For drug users, Dilaudid helped avoid dopesickness and reduce our reliance on the street supply. *Crackdown* talked to a sex worker who was able to turn down the most risky dates because of her Dilly script. But the drug supply continued to get worse and worse. People got wired to a harrowing mix of fentanyl, benzos, xylazine, nitazenes and other shit that was in the street supply. Dilaudid just can't substitute for all that. So some resorted to selling their prescribed Dilaudid to afford the illicit down they were wired to. Mostly they were selling to other people with experience of opioid use, like me. Research from Professors Thomas Kerr and Geoff Bardwell confirmed that, in the context of the deadly, contaminated illicit supply, this kind of "diversion" was often saving people's lives. I was able to avoid street down because I could buy Dilaudid from friends with prescriptions. I am very grateful for this. But we didn't call it diversion. We called it sharing.

When I was coming up, I learned a street code. It included principles like never introducing anyone new to heroin and never leaving rigs around where they could stick someone. There was also a respect for children in the code. When you see a family with children walking down the street, call out "kids on the block" to warn everyone ahead. Then people stop smoking rock or dealing or whatever sketchy activity they might be up to. "Goof" was also the worst insult. It means "child abuser," and illustrates how much contempt drug users have for anyone who hurts children. Many of us were harmed when we were young, so we take it seriously.

A few months after Global aired its Dilaudid story, BCAPOM coordinator Hannah Dempsey was struggling with the big TV at the front of VANDU's main room. She told everyone that the wait would be worth it: "You'll want to see this." She finally got it to work.

"With controversy raging," said another Global newscaster,

"we hit the streets of Vancouver Friday to find out what was really happening."

The story's journalist, Paul Johnson, appeared onscreen, instantly causing the room to burst with laughter. For some reason, Johnson had decided to go undercover. He wore a black ball cap, a graphic T-shirt and cheap-looking sunglasses. Johnson explained that he was going to prove that it was possible to buy Dilaudid on the street—the same Dilaudid that doctors were prescribing through the risk mitigation program.

At Main and Hastings, which we all knew as "Pill Corner," Johnson held up a zip-lock bag containing twenty-six Dilaudid pills that he explained he'd just bought from one of the dealers.

"What kind of *news* is this?" someone asked.

Everyone mumbled in agreement. For most people in the room, twenty-six Dillies would be breakfast. And, since the early 1990s, well before the risk mitigation program started, everybody knew that you could buy diverted meds on Pill Corner. There had always been Dilaudid there. The cops knew about Pill Corner as well, but they hardly ever did anything about it. Nevertheless, the Global piece had a "gotcha" tone.

More snickers erupted when, at the end of the piece, Johnson, still in costume, strolled into a police station to turn the pills over to the cops. "Will they even care about that?" someone asked. In a different political environment, Johnson's story would have faded off into harmless obscurity. After all, for an investigative piece, it revealed practically nothing at all. How often were risk mitigation patients diverting their meds? Were the diverted pills having a mostly helpful or mostly harmful impact on the overdose crisis? *Why* were some people diverting the medication instead of taking it themselves? And why were others buying diverted medication instead of simply getting it from a doctor? Johnson didn't say. The piece never even conclusively proved that the twenty-six pills had come from the risk mitigation program at all. But in the context of Poilievre's moral panic around "woke" government drugs, this kind of rigour and detail was no longer necessary.

In April, I was invited to be part of a panel at the Canadian Association of Journalists conference. The panel was about reporting on the overdose crisis. I told the assembled reporters that a moral panic was brewing and that the news media was playing a major role. A silent room looked back at me. I pleaded with them: Please don't be part of the backlash this time. Don't let the right spread lies and slander totally unchecked. Programs will be shut down. People will die. But I got blank stares and crickets.

In June 2023, my government sources told me that a group of clinicians had met with Premier Eby to tell him they were worried about the risk mitigation program. The doctors had seen the news stories and were upset. They wanted Eby to cancel the program altogether. And—according to my sources— Eby was strongly considering their request.

It was a big decision. If Eby cancelled RMG outright, it would have been his most direct and provocative salvo against the drug user movement to date. It would also be a gift to his political opponents, read as an admission of defeat—as evidence that Poilievre had been right all along. At the time, the NDP still had a decent lead in the polls. But Poilievre had effectively stained the Dilly program, and the government needed to decide: Do we distance ourselves from this or do we defend it?

BC's provincial health officer, Dr. Bonnie Henry, convinced Eby to hold off for the time being. She announced that she would be reviewing the program and would share her results with the people of BC. Studies had shown the life-saving outcomes of the program. But it didn't matter. An avalanche of columns, articles, TV news pieces and speeches in the House of Commons continued to spread disinformation and fear about safe supply. A few courageous doctors were hounded online. Hundreds of people had their Dilaudid prescriptions cut off. And it continues.

Amidst the backlash, Eby started to equivocate about decriminalization as well. Since day one, right-wing politicians had blamed BCs decriminalization pilot program for causing a spike in public drug use, even though there was no evidence that public drug use had increased under the new rules. In fact, VPD inspector Phil Heard would later admit that public complaints about drug users had actually *decreased* under decriminalization—an inconvenient fact that the VPD had kept quiet until it was too late for the information to be useful. Nevertheless, in news story after news story, police complained that they now had "no tools" to stop people from using drugs—even when they were near a family on the beach or in a restaurant. A video of patrons smoking something in a Tim Hortons went viral, and BC's conservative politicians threw a fit in the legislature.

The outrage about decriminalization was smart political theatre. Pundits blamed long-standing social problems on the new policy. It seemed to me that the cops were choosing to stand down more and more in situations where they could easily intervene. Like a kind of secret strike. Of course, the truth was that cops had plenty of tools to stop public drug use. It was illegal to smoke *anything* inside a restaurant. And the decriminalization policy already included a list of exempted places—such as playgrounds and schools—where it was illegal to possess drugs. The cops could still arrest people for intoxication, mischief or causing a disturbance. I had still seen cops stopping and searching people. I was standing on the corner of Hastings and Gore when a cop told me to move along.

The BC NDP responded to the complaints first by issuing a press release announcing new "measures to ensure families feel safe accessing public spaces." It had a picture of three children blowing bubbles on a sunny day. The message was clear: the very sight of drug users is a danger to the young. VANDU members had become pretty numb to insults from the government, but that one stung. In meeting after meeting, our members talked about how much they loved their own children. I thought of Paige. The government was acting like we were monsters.

Reading the press release again, I noticed the precise use of language. The phrase "feel safe" was used several times. The government was careful not to say that anybody was in real danger, and it didn't cite any statistics or examples. But their press release acknowledged the growing *feeling* of unease in the air. And it promised that the BC NDP would be taking that feeling seriously.

The government could have defended decriminalization. They could have told the public that during the first eight months of decrim, possession offences were down 77 per cent. They could have brought one of us to a press conference to talk about how a possession charge had derailed our lives. They could have spoken about the racist origin of these laws, or about the way the laws were still used disproportionately against Black and Indigenous people. They could have explained that public drug use had not increased. But instead, they folded like a cheap tent.

Standing at a podium on April 26, 2024, Eby announced he was requesting the federal government recriminalize the simple possession of drugs everywhere in the province except for at supervised consumption sites (where drugs were already allowed) and in private residences (where the cops seldom made possession busts anyway). Drug users would be forced back to the alleys and to the shadows. Eby admitted, "There's no question that criminalizing drug use costs all of us. It costs threats to lives. It costs money for prosecutions, and it doesn't make us safer." But he did it nonetheless. It was a crass political calculation. Eby and the NDP didn't want to be defending decriminalization during the coming election campaign.

The feds quickly approved Eby's request, effectively gutting the program. In the House of Commons, Poilievre celebrated the decision as a big win for the Canadian right. Eby's capitulation— Poilievre argued—was proof that decriminalization leads naturally to disorder and chaos. And that this would happen wherever and whenever decriminalization was tried. Across the country, the media ran Poilievre's claims more or less unchallenged, almost never mentioning that public drug use had not *actually* increased during the decrim pilot. Or that public drug use occurs in cities outside of BC, where decriminalization was never tried. The BC NDP had, yet again, managed to tarnish one of our good ideas on the global stage.

"In Canada, we had 115 years of prohibition," I said on *Crackdown*. "And only fifteen months to try decrim. So they had over a century, and their thing failed again and again. And we had fifteen months to try ours. And it *was* showing some good results." I argued that Eby's cowardice would ultimately come back to haunt him. And as the right consolidated its grip on the electorate, the BC NDP started to slip in the polls.

We knew it was just a matter of time before the backlash came for VANDU and DULF directly. The campaign was led by the shadow minister for addictions, Elenore Sturko. Sturko was part of the right-leaning BC United party but would later switch to the further-right Conservative Party of British Columbia. She was also a former sergeant with the Surrey RCMP and a recovered alcoholic. Sturko explained to reporters that she started to drink two bottles of wine a night to cope with the PTSD she'd gotten on the job. Sturko fought for tough sentences for dealers and involuntary treatment for drug users. In many ways, Sturko was a throwback to the 1980s-style drug war of Ronald and Nancy Reagan.

But nothing seemed to bother Sturko quite like DULF. "Just because we're in the midst of a crisis," Sturko told reporters, "doesn't mean that we have to suddenly throw away the rule of law in British Columbia." It was our publicness, our brazenness, that singled us out for retaliation. Sturko did her best to paint DULF's compassionate giveaways as something far more sinister, arguing that because we had bought drugs from the dark web, we were contributing to a funding stream for human trafficking, illegal weapons and terrorism. It was a ludicrous argument. Terrible things happened in every corner of the internet. Facebook's algorithms had been accused of facilitating a genocide against the Rohingya—was everyone with an FB account supporting the war crime? Obviously not.

Sturko demanded that BC's attorney general conduct a forensic audit into DULF and VANDU to see if any government or research funds had gone toward drugs. But DULF had been careful, using only private donations to purchase drugs. Funds from the Vancouver Coastal Health Authority had been put toward the cost of running DULF's overdose prevention site and the rent on its small Downtown Eastside storefront. Nonetheless, Sturko was able to convince the government to cut its funding to DULF. I worried VANDU would be next.

Three weeks later, the VPD raided DULF's storefront as well as Eris's and Jeremy's apartments. The cops seized the organization's drugs and money and, later, arrested Eris and Jeremy, eventually charging them each with three counts of possession for the purposes of trafficking. It had taken three and a half years for the state to finally smash DULF. But we aren't going quietly. Eris and Jeremy's defence counsel will seek to challenge the legal underpinnings of drug prohibition in the highest court of the land. The drug war itself could be on trial.

One week later, the BC Coroners Service released its *Death Review Panel*. The report, which was convened by chief coroner Lisa Lapointe, called on the province to "immediately pursue" expanded access to safer supply, including through non-medicalized models. "Safer supply is not a radical initiative," Lapointe argued. "It's a means to keep people alive and to support them to wellness. It's a means to reduce our loved ones' dependency on a toxic, profit-driven, illicit drug market. It is a life support." When reporters asked Lapointe about DULF, she told them, "I suppose I would say that if you see somebody in a burning house, you feel somewhat justified to smash the window."

I went to visit my friend Howard to see how he was doing. I knew he'd probably be sitting with his dog, Iffin, on his stoop across from the park. Howard was the very first member of DULF's compassion club. For decades, he'd used opioids to deal with a painful autoimmune disease. It was only after getting a spot in DULF's compassion club—and after receiving a Dilaudid prescription from the RMG program—that Howard was able to keep himself away from the toxic drug supply. Now, without the DULF compassion club, I worried that he was in danger.

"How are you doing, man? What are you gonna do now?" I asked.

"I don't know, Garth," he said, patting his dog. "I really don't know."

"Do you have any kind of plan or anything?"

Howard stared straight ahead for a while. He looked helpless. I tried my best to think of something to say—to give him hope. But I couldn't come up with anything. Howard and I both knew his survival would be in question.

———

It may look like our enemies are winning. Prohibition started amidst a racist panic more than a century ago. Canada spent decades punishing and banishing people. But drugs today are more potent and more common than ever. Everyone can see it. Today's backlash is just the most recent in a long history of moral panics. The drug warriors aren't actually winning. They're desperate. We've been chipping away at prohibition for years, and it's starting to crumble. We aren't hearing their triumphant battle cry. We're hearing the death rattle of the drug war—but like a wounded animal, its proponents are dangerous.

Their dream of a drug-free world has never been possible. Humans have always used substances for ceremony, to manage pain, to escape boredom or to unwind. Many of us use drugs to momentarily fill the holes in our ruined hearts, to duct-tape our broken lives. Drugs can temporarily stop flashbacks of a chaotic childhood or replace a mother's love never known. Drugs can hit the pause button on the pain, guilt, self-hate and fear of our present. Drugs can provide a bit of shelter.

We numb ourselves from all kinds of wounds—poverty, colonization, violence, the drudgery of work, the terror of homelessness, the brutality of racism, homophobia and transphobia, injuries we got on the job, childhood abuse or that grinding feeling of powerlessness.

And when dopesickness returns, all that pain held momentarily at bay comes crashing back down upon us, threatening to drown us. So we go out and score—taking our lives into our own hands—and try to get well. But we're made criminals for it and are cast out.

Our dead are beyond counting. We're angry because none of this needed to happen. Like Laura told me, "If the government ever gets around to fixing this, there won't be any of us left."

I don't know if it was Jeff telling me to, or just a little voice inside me, but I decided to come clean. I asked Lisa to go for a walk, and we wandered over to the train tracks. We sat on a bench, and I told her that I hadn't been totally honest lately.

"I've been chipping," I said. "Taking Dillies on top of the methadone." I didn't have any excuses. There had been no reason to lie. And I felt awful about it. "I'm sorry," I said. "I thought I had left this kind of thing behind. I was just worried you'd leave."

"No. I'm not going anywhere," Lisa said. "I knew you were burnt out and sad. I think we were so focused on making sure I didn't lose my shit that we didn't take care of you. I'm just glad there was something you could use that wasn't the contaminated crap on the street. I don't wanna lose you."

"Things have been pretty fucked up," I explained—knowing full well that this wouldn't be news to her. "After we lost the babies, and everybody kept dying . . . I just couldn't take it."

Lisa put her head on my shoulder, and we sat on the bench as the sun got lower in the sky. "We're in this for the long haul," she said.

I raised my methadone dose, quit the Dillies and started sessions with Dr. Joanne again, unravelling the ball of grief and pain that had tangled up my life. After one of those sessions, I called my parents. I told them about Victoria. They said they'd have done things differently if they'd known. I hung up and went to find Lisa. "They believed me, they actually believed me," I told her.

A Warm Blanket

The years of the backlash were among the hardest years of the crisis. Elections loomed on the horizon. A new crowd of right-wing leaders was rising up, and we had to steel ourselves for the fights ahead. But one day in late August came as a great relief. Jeff and I joined about fifty other VANDU members who were gathering in Oppenheimer Park on International Overdose Awareness Day. It was a warm evening, and some people were sitting on the grass. I said hello to a few friends and comrades. Most voices seemed subdued. I walked over to look at a stack of blankets laid out carefully on the grass. Each had a stunning pattern of repeating stars. Delilah saw me looking at the blankets. She was the last of the "Fab Four" Indigenous women who led VANDU. The other three—Chereece Keewatin, Tracey Morrison and Flora Munroe—had all died of overdose over the last several years. Delilah said, "We've been sewing these for the past twelve months." The Western Aboriginal Harm Reduction Society had been planning and preparing for this ceremony for a long time. As a non-Indigenous person, I felt humbled that I was invited to be a part of it.

In the weeks before, Hannah and Elder Kelly White invited

VANDU members to put forward the names of friends and family who had died over the last few years. We would stand in for them, and they would be blanketed posthumously. It had been a few years since my friend Wade had died. I knew his family back in Six Nations was missing him, and they would be moved by this ceremony, so I put his name forward. Jeff put forward his old friend Otis, who had died around the same time as Wade.

At the park, Hannah guided us all to stand in a large circle around the star blankets. An eagle flew in big loops high overhead. Carleen Thomas from Tsleil-Waututh, Mary Point from Musqueam and Kelly White from Snuneymuxw presided over the ceremony. "This is called K'emk'emeláy," Kelly said, gesturing to the city around us, "which means place of many maple trees." She explained that the blanketing ceremony we were about to do is a traditional Indigenous practice symbolizing protection, respect and healing. Kelly made her way around the inside of the circle. She stopped at each person to fan them with sage and sweetgrass smoke, using an eagle feather. One by one, each decedent's name was called. And one by one, Hannah escorted each of us to the centre of the circle in the quiet park. I heard name after name. I had known almost every single one. Our circle represented so much loss. The pressure built up in my chest and throat. I thought about all the funerals, all the trips to Glenhaven Memorial Chapel and everyone who was already gone.

Then Carleen called Wade's name. Hannah ushered me to the centre. I thought about what a sharing guy Wade was. I remembered this one time he offered to give me his Johnny

Cash T-shirt. I love Johnny Cash, but I knew Wade didn't have many shirts, so I declined. I'd always wondered if I'd hurt Wade by refusing his gift.

Carleen and Kelly said a few words and wrapped a purple-and-pink star blanket around my shoulders and pinned it at the chest. All the grief I had been choking back, forcing down and numbing out with Dilaudid flowed out freely. I cried. Everyone's eyes were shiny with tears. Hannah walked me to the far side of the circle, where I took my place with the others who already had blankets around them.

After the ceremony, Jeff and I sat on the grass with Hannah, Delilah, Samona and Laura. The ceremony had taken a lot of energy. We felt tired but happy. We talked quietly and ate hot dogs as the sun went down. I felt as light as Kelly's eagle feather.

I thought of all my comrades in the movement and all the people I grew up with. I had been losing people most of my life. I'd been to many more memorials than weddings or baby showers. The loss isn't just confined to Vancouver. Across the country, there are people missing from factories, offices, churches, universities, building sites, bands, gurdwaras, community centres and family gatherings. We are everywhere, and it'll just keep happening until something changes.

All the drug users, people in recovery, activists, students, academics, journalists, and parents—we'd all taken different paths to get here, but we were united in a shared experience: each of us was unable to stomach the violence of the drug war. We'd all taken on personal risk to help others. We were a family joined by a commitment to love and solidarity.

A series of faces flashed in my mind. Nick, Wade, Chereece, Tracey, Flora, Janis, Greg, Dave. It suddenly felt like they were there with us too. Just for a moment. And I hoped that they were resting easy, safe in the knowledge that we are carrying on their work. And eventually we will win.

Acknowledgements

I wrote this book on Musqueam, Squamish and Tsleil-Waututh territory.

Joe Strummer once said, "Without people, you're nothing." This is so true for me, and without my people, this book wouldn't exist. When we met, my wife, Lisa Hale, said, "There's a book in you." She helped get it out of me and was with me for every step. I love you. My oldest friend and brother, Jeff Louden, told me to keep it simple. My friend, bandmate and *Crackdown* podcast Senior Producer, Sam Fenn, applied his story-structure magic. Ward Hawkes at Doubleday Canada edited the book, along with Sam and Lisa. When the publisher first reached out, neighbour and author Ryan Knighton showed me the ropes. Thanks to Laura Shaver, who taught me how to let go of shame and tell my story. Thanks also to my agent Christopher Schelling of Selectric Artists.

Thanks to Lisa and all of my family, especially my parents, Gary and Doreen Mullins, my niece Nym, who once went by the name Paige, and to my great grandmother Rosa Mullins, who spent twenty-six years locked up in Riverview Mental Hospital and told them, "You will not destroy me." Thanks to my late grandfather Ted Mullins for teaching me shortwave radio, basic electronics and advanced curiosity, and to Rose Magdalena Moifong Wilking, my late great-aunt, who brought our family together with food and love.

Thanks to the *Crackdown* podcast Editorial Board: Dean Wilson, the elder statesman of our movement, who is pictured on the cover, Samona Marsh, Reija Jean, Laura Shaver, Shelda Kastor, Jeff Louden, Martin Steward, Elli Taylor, Delilah Gregg and members who have passed on: Chereece Keewatin, Dave Murray and Greg Fresz. Thanks to *Crackdown* Producers Sam Fenn, Alexander B. Kim, Alex de Boer and Lisa Hale. Thanks to academic collaborators Ryan McNeil, Jade Boyd, Susan Boyd, Thomas Kerr, Danya Fast, Rebecca Haines-Saah, Andrea Lopez and Peter Klein. Thanks to everyone who's listened to and supported the *Crackdown* podcast.

Thanks, VANDU, BCAPOM & WAHRS leaders Lorna Bird, Hugh Lampkin, Dave Hamm, Jon Braithwaite, JJ, Ryan Maddeaux and Kelly White. Thanks to past & present VANDU organizers Brittany Graham, Vince Tao, Hannah Dempsey, Aiyanas Ormond, Aaron Bailey, Nate Compton and Ann Livingston.

Thanks to bandmates Steve Schramel, Geoff Cousins (RIP), Matt Bruce, Kai Paulson, Mike Ray, James Ash, Ray Garraway (RIP), Jay Hehn, Mikey Bowd, Derek Simpson, Errol Prince, Andy, Sam and others for putting up with my utilitarian guitar playing.

Thanks for helping me recall the past, Erica Elana Berman, Natasha Hambiln, Lauren Goff, Tracey Helton Mitchell, Michael Assouline and historian Lani Russwurm.

Thanks to Dr. M for prescribing methadone and to Dr. Joanne for treating my PTSD. Thanks to Simon, Gurj, Kim, Michelle and everyone for all the help and care over the years.

Thanks to friends and comrades: Tonye Aganaba, Meenakshi Manno, Jaggi Singh, Caitlin Shane, Jason Gratl, Cameron Ward, Tim Dickson, Tyson Singh Kelsall, Alissa Westergard-Thorpe, Jagdeep Singh Mangat (RIP), Petra Shulz, Leslie McBain, everyone at Moms Stop the Harm, Nicole Luongo, Shane Calder, Matt Bonn, Corey Ranger, Beverly Ho, Otis Rotting, Brian McDougal, Harsha Walia, Donald MacPherson, Zool & Zak Suleman, Ryan Suds, Tony Tracy, Kamuran Sadar, Saul Schneider, Charles Boylan (RIP), Guy Felicella, Sid Tan, Gabrielle Peters, Anmol Swaich, Eris Nyx, Jeremy Kalicum, everyone at DULF, Sharmeen Khan, Ikponwosa "IK" Ero, Hawkfeather, Isin Can and Peter Ash. Thanks to brother Grand Chief Doug Kelly and Carleen Thomas.

Thanks to all harm reduction workers and drug user movement organizers everywhere. Thanks to everyone in the labour movement fighting for workers.

Thanks to journalists Andrea Woo, Zachary Seigel, Rumneek Johal, Derrick O'Keefe, Greg Kelley, Yvonne Gall, Stephen Quinn and Euan Thompson.

Gone too soon: Bronwyn Charmin, Fiona Munro, Tracey Morrison, Wade Crawford, Ron Kuhlke, Crystal Boudreau, Jeremy the Amoeba, Dixie Dugan, Janis Warren, Lori Preston, Bud Osborn, Charlie Boyle, John Turvey, TJ & Dylan, Kurt, Noel and so many more.

Love to the cats Shadow, Shaggy, Stumbles and Salvador. We miss you so much.